MISSION
CHIROPRACTIC

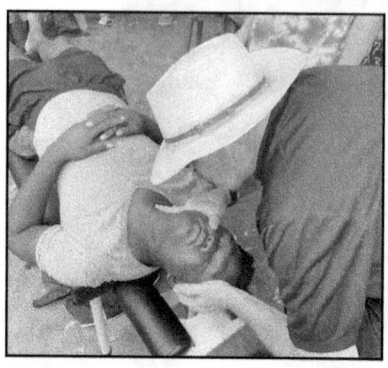

Adjusting session during the mission

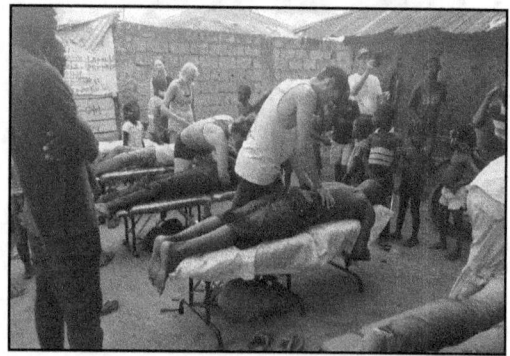

Labadee, Haiti. Named after Marquis de La Badie, a French slave owner who settled here in the 1600's. His descendants fought against Henri Christopher and his army of former black slaves.

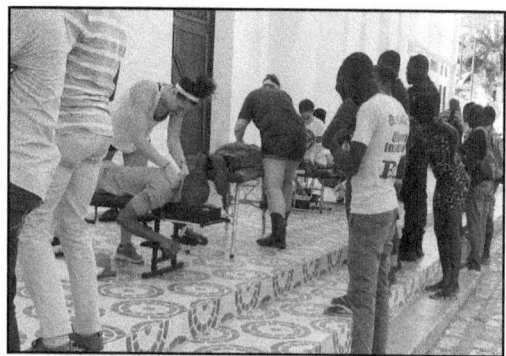

We are in front of the Cathedral Notre-Dame in Cap-Hatian. Cathedral dates from 1670. In the square of the cathedral the liberation of the slaves was proclaimed August 29, 1793.

MISSION CHIROPRACTIC

Changing the World By Touching Lives

PETER MORGAN, DC

Mission Chiropractic
Copyright © 2020 by Peter Morgan, DC
All rights reserved.

No part of this publication may be reproduced, distributed, or transmitted in any form or by any means, including photocopying, recording, or other electronic or mechanical methods, without the prior written permission of the author, except in the case of brief quotations embodied in critical reviews and certain other noncommercial uses permitted by copyright law.

ISBN (paperback): 978-1-7353184-0-0
ISBN (hardcover): 978-1-7353184-4-8
ISBN (ebook): 978-1-7353184-1-7

All content contained herein was originally written by Peter Morgan, DC, with the exception of personal stories contributed by others and shared with permission. Portions of the contents of this book have been previously published. Such material has been edited and is reprinted here with permission from Dr. Morgan. Original sources include *The 5-Day Missionary* (Peter Morgan, 2020) and *The Chiropractic Journal* (April 2007, March 2008, June 2008, July 2009, November 2009, January 2010, March 2010, June 2010, March 2011, June 2011, December 2011, March 2012, June 2015).

Website: https://www.missionlifeinternational.com/

Printed in the United States of America

This book is dedicated to the more than three thousand chiropractors who have attended one of the nearly one hundred chiropractic mission trips I have led through Mission Life International Foundation. I pray that our missions have inspired all of you to be great chiropractors.

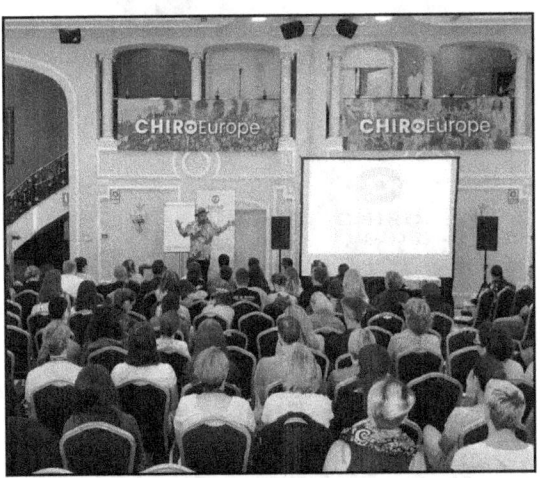

ChiroEurope 2018

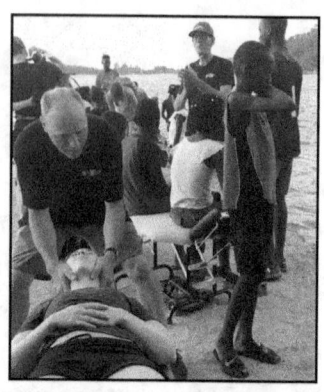

At a small fishing village on the coast of Haiti with Dr. Gille from Quebec.

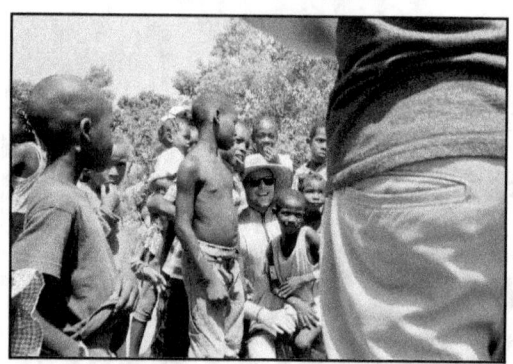

Michael Dibley, DC sharing Chiropractic.

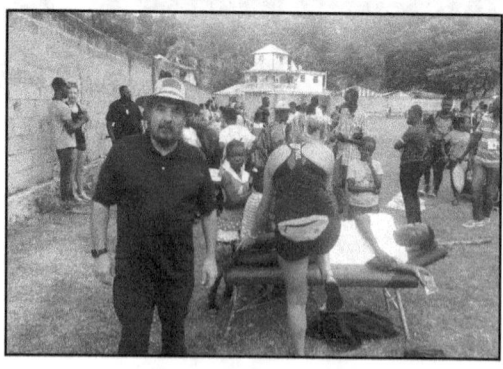

Inside a soccer stadium in Labadee, Haiti.

Contents

Foreword   xi

Introduction: From Chiropractor to Mission Leader   1

PART I: The Chiropractic Mission   7

1. The Philosophy, Science, and Art of Chiropractic   9
2. Chiropractic Humanitarians   23
3. Mission Chiropractic   33
4. Innate Intelligence   39
5. Joy and Serenity through Service   49
6. Your Chiropractic Mission   55

PART II: The Mission Experience   65
7. The Impact of Chiropractic Mission Trips   67
8. My First Chiropractic Mission Trip, 9/11   71
9. Mission Trip to Dominican Republic, March 2007   87
10. Mission Trip to Haiti, April 2008   93
11. Mission Trip to Haiti, June 2008   101
12. Mission Trip to Dominican Republic and Haiti, October 2008   109
13. Mission Trip to Cuba, January 2010   121
14. Haiti Earthquake 2010   129

15. One Year after the Earthquake	137
16. Mission Trip to Haiti and Dominican Republic, February 2012	143
17. Mission Trip to Haiti and Dominican Republic, March 2012	151
18. Mission Trip to Dominican Republic, October 2012	157
19. World Record Mission Trip to Haiti, January 2013	163
20. The United Nations Military Base, Haiti, April 2013	169
21. Mission Trip to Haiti, March 2018	173
APPENDIX: Mission Statements	179

MY MISSION STATEMENT

I am committed to a special vision. DD Palmers vision. I envision a world free of nerve interference, through the correction of vertebral subluxations for the best expression of each person's human potential. I am committed to serving all people with chiropractic care throughout their lifetime. I will travel all over the world to serve Man's greatest gift to man "Chiropractic"

I acknowledge that vertebral subluxations and interference to the meninges are a serious insult to the nerve system. I am committed to educating each person to the benefits of chiropractic care for the correction of vertebral subluxations and restoration and maintenance of optimal health throughout their lifetime.

My mission is to serve my community and to serve people in developing nations with quality health care and to direct people to the realization that health comes from within, and ultimately that the maintenance of health is superior to the treatment of disease. I encourage each person to participate in this most important and noble mission.

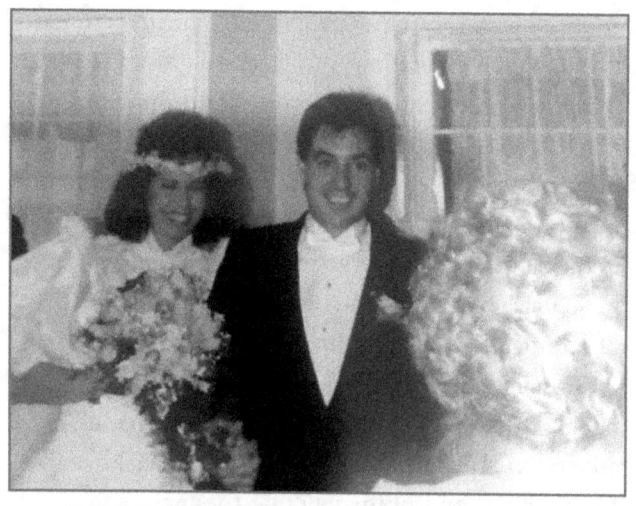

On July 2, 1988 I married my best friend and soulmate.
Love you Theresa.

FOREWORD

Whenever I think about my profession of chiropractic; I think about it's great chiropractic leaders. DD Palmer, BJ Palmer, Frank DiGiacomo, Sid Williams and the many others who have moved chiropractic's growth and development in a positive direction. I first met Dr. Peter Morgan at New York Chiropractic College in 1982, and I could tell right away there was something uniquely different about him. He had this contagious energy and unrelenting enthusiasm for life that attracted you to him like a magnet. He had just returned to the U.S. from attending medical school in Italy, and it wasn't long before we became roommates in a Frat-style house on a beach in Bayville, NY.

An era of incredible chiropractic education, camaraderie, stormy episodes and challenges. One thing about Peter, he did everything at 110%. Whether it be work or play, he always went ALL OUT! I remember one time we were playing tackle football with some of the biggest most physical guys in the school. Peter was the smallest contestant on the field but played with such hustle that after only fifteen minutes into the game,

NO ONE wanted to be tackled by him—they would purposely just take a dive to avoid the savage ferocity he would unleash. It was like getting hit by a cannon, which earned him the name "Pistol Pete"—a name he has lived up to, to this day.

This unrelenting passion and zest for life has carried over into his professional career as he has blazed trails in chiropractic that have never before been forged. Peter is an expression of the "big idea". His innate leadership abilities became evident early on in his career. He became president of the New York Chiropractic Council and in 2001 was named chiropractor of the year. Over the years he has been presented with numerous humanitarian awards. He was among the first group of chiropractors on the scene during 911. His organization was leading the charge and mobilizing convoys of DC's to Ground Zero to treat all the first responders during that horrific crisis.

Subsequently, Peter organized and pioneered mission trips to third world countries like Trinidad, Tobago, Cuba, the Bahamas, the Dominican Republic and Haiti. He was one of the first to open chiropractic offices in those deprived areas and brought chiropractic forward to the world in places that had never before experienced a chiropractic adjustment. He was one of the first Americans to return to Haiti after the devastating earthquake of 2010, to provide aid and mobilize relief efforts in that demolished and ravaged country. Peter led over 60 mission trips to Haiti post earthquake, raising money to build a school and an orphanage for all of the children who had lost their parents in the devastation. He has completed 98 mission trips to date and is returning to Haiti with another mission in August 2020. His unyielding devotion to chiropractic has elevated him to one of the unsung heroes of our profession—but it's his selfless dedication to humanity that is the essence of what he truly represents.

I am a great admirer of Dr. Peter Morgan and can honestly say that he is one of the most genuine individuals I have ever met. This book exemplifies his perseverance and "Commitment to the cause" and embodies the authentic nature of his character. I am truly honored to call him my friend.

I love you brother—you make me proud!

Adam Deltorto, DC

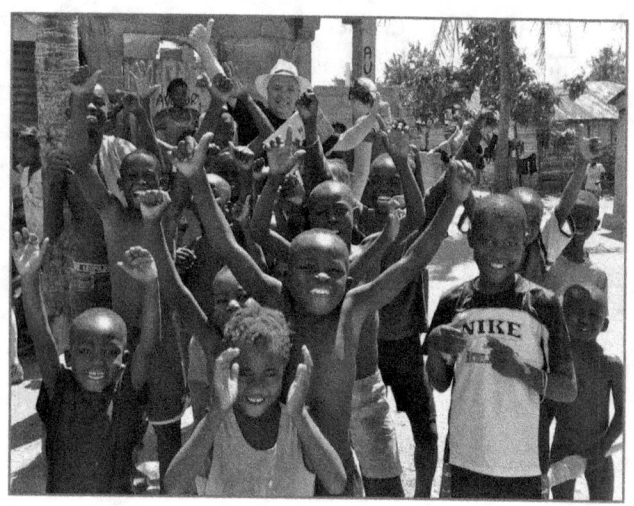

Ouanaminthe, Haiti 2011

INTRODUCTION

From Chiropractor to Mission Leader

Taking care of injured people was always a dream of mine. Chiropractic is a holistic, natural, hands-on healing profession, and I am now a traditional chiropractor. I practiced chiropractic for many years, built a huge chiropractic office, and helped many injured people. I bought a nice home in an affluent area thirty-five minutes from midtown Manhattan. As my chiropractic practice grew, so did my stress. I was always busy taking care of people with many types of injuries—auto injuries, work injuries, slip-and-falls, sports injuries, and construction injuries.

I felt that everyone wanted something from me. Lawyers wanted narratives and extensive notes, and wanted me to go to court to testify, among other such things. I loved taking care of people, but I did not feel an inner sense of joy and serenity. I was dissatisfied, and felt that I was just working to try to meet my expenses. I was too concerned with the collections.

Eventually, I realized that something was missing. I knew my purpose was helping injured people and that it was a good purpose, but something was missing. What was my true purpose in life? What was my mission in life? What was my purpose for my existence in this universe? I kept feeling that I had not done enough for my fellow man.

A good friend of mine mentioned that a great seminar for chiropractors was coming, so I went. I listened to a speaker named Pasquale Cerasoli, DC. Shortly after the seminar, I had a lucid dream. I dreamed that I was with Jesus and D.D. Palmer, the founder of chiropractic. The dream was very spiritual. In it, Jesus revealed my path as a missionary, and D.D. instructed me on the ways of chiropractic. As the dream concluded, I made a solemn oath that I would bring forth this spiritual message. I would lead and teach students and the public about becoming a missionary.

This incredible dream was a revelation that chiropractic could reunite the physical with the spiritual. As the dream was concluding, I made a solemn oath to Palmer that I would bring forth this spiritual message of chiropractic. I would lead and teach chiropractors, students, and the public about chiropractic. I would help to lead this great profession to glory.

Before this dream, I was a chiropractor. Since this dream, I have been a chiropractic leader and spiritual missionary. I began studying philosophy, theology, and spiritualism. I started going to bible classes, and read the works of Mother Teresa, who said that God will judge us on how we loved and how much compassion we had for our brother and sisters. She said that God comes to us in the "distressing disguise of the poor" and asks us for our help. I understood this to mean that the universe wants us to fill our spirit with love; with compassion, we serve our fellow man with kindness, joy, and the love and compassion of angels. In order to have spiritual growth, we need to serve love and compassion to all humanity. Our mission must be to alleviate the suffering of others, especially the poor.

A few months after my lucid dream, I encountered my longtime friend Dr. Todd Herold. While talking with him, we decided to create chiropractic mission trips. I already had been attending mission trips with my church since 2002. In 1980 I lived in a monastery in Perugia, Italy. Incredibly, I assisted clergy from the Monteripido monastery in attending to those who were injured during the 6.9 earthquake that centered in the village of Potenza.

Todd and I wanted to help as many people in developing countries as possible. As we discussed our dream, we learned that a colleague, chiropractor JC Doornick, had recently been denied a Doctors without Borders trip because the organization allows only those in the allopathic profession. They do not allow chiropractors.

JC also had the vision of bringing natural health care to poor and developing countries. Together we decided to create a chiropractic mission to Dominican

Republic. During that time, I had a spiritual journey, and I discovered my mission and purpose in life. My spiritual transformation required a commitment and a willingness to lose some close friends and even family members. My associates were perplexed. Some thought that I was nutty, crazy, confused, and bewildered. However, once I undertook this journey, I was filled with unconditional love and compassion. It enabled me to find serenity and joy. Most importantly, I discovered my mission in life.

In 2002 I founded Chiromissions, an organization that organizes chiropractic mission trips. In January 2010 I founded Mission Life International Foundation, a charitable organization that operates the Mission Life Family Orphanage. This organization also works with Chiromissions to organize mission trips. To this day I lead from four to eight mission trips every year, and over three thousand people have served some of the world's poorest people through these missions. Mission Life International is a charitable organization with 501(c)3 status. All funds donated to Mission Life International are tax deductible for US citizens.

We need a cultural shift, a changing paradigm, to take place for a better world, one that will alter our world in a beneficial way, one that places attention and value on the individual's spirituality.

I acknowledge that God is the all-pervading, ecumenical intelligence. I state unequivocally that there is a universal intelligence. Every person is a consciousness that is a quantum part of this universal intelligence in a dual entity of the physical and spiritual. The spirit is a quantum spirit. In the physical, the quantum spirit is in every cell. This is part of the intelligent, creative principle.

Every person is called upon for service, but only some answer. Those who do answer encounter the greatest riches in the universe. The information presented here is intended to provide you with a road map to your calling, the course to your purpose and your mission. Your service is very important and needed by many.

If your mission is chiropractic, then the information contained in this book will show you the benefits of walking the talk of mission chiropractic.

PRAYER FOR MY PURPOSE

Thank you, God, for providing me with my purpose, my mission, my destiny. I affirm the power of my healing energy expressed through my healing hands. I affirm that I am a vehicle for bringing light to the people of the world. I am blessed to be one of those chosen to bring your healing energy to people who are suffering with afflictions.

Through your gift, I have the power to tune up the nervous systems of thousands of people. Thank you for the enlightenment that the relationship between man and universal intelligence is a direct one. The avenue that the mind of the universe expresses to the mind of man is through the innate intelligence of man himself. I am that I am.

My practice members are blessed to meet me because of the divine qualities that I am offering. Those divine qualities are your power, God, through me. We chiropractors are God in action on Earth, expressing the divine power through our healing hands. All that I need, I have. All that I desire is mine as I give thanks and share these healing hands with love and joy.

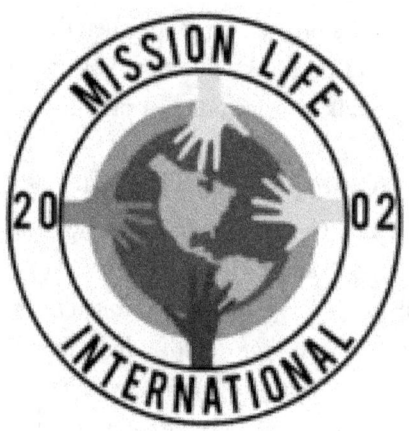

Our logo signifies that we are changing the world by touching lives.

PART I

The Chiropractic Mission

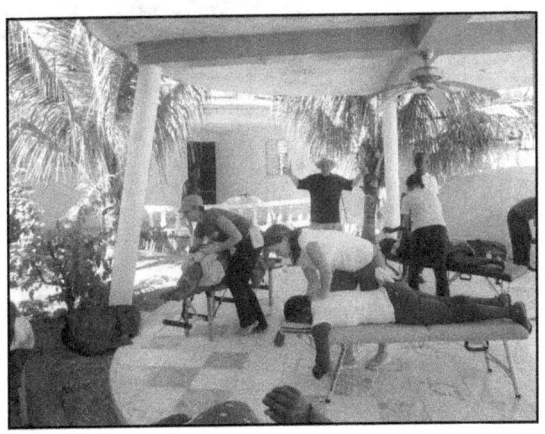

Dominican Republic 2012.

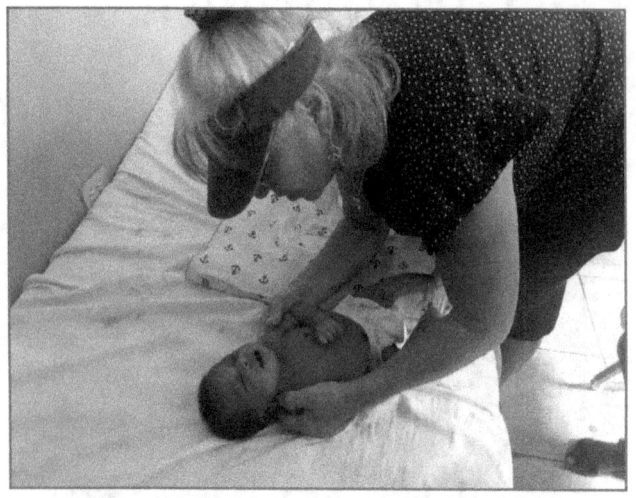

Dr. Patti Giuliano adjusting an infant.

CHAPTER 1

The Philosophy, Science, and Art of Chiropractic

You must give some time to your fellow men. Even if it's a little thing, do something for others, something for which you get no pay but the privilege of doing it.

—ALBERT SCHWEITZER

Chiropractic is a philosophy, a science, and an art. The philosophy of chiropractic expresses the wisdom postulated by the thirty-three principles of chiropractic that constitute the science of chiropractic.

Chiropractic art consists of the science of utilizing the spinous and transverse processes of the neuroskeleton as levers to tune up the nervous system. The art of chiropractic has to do with the correct kinesiology of the vertebrae.

Science is a system of knowledge that covers the operation of generalized laws. Chiropractic is the name of a classified, indexed knowledge of sequential sense impressions of biology. It is the science of life that is expressed in Ralph W. Stephenson's "33 Chiropractic Principles," published in his 1927 *Chiropractic Textbook*. Chiropractors must know not only the basic principle on which chiropractic is based and the intrinsic parts that construct its scientific design, but also the philosophy of the science and art of adjusting the neuroskeleton.

If our mission is chiropractic, then we must study and comprehend chiropractic science and these thirty-three principles. We must live by these principles so that we can develop new and perhaps better methods in adjusting subluxated vertebrae and cranial facial bones.

The objectives of a chiropractic education should be the acquisition of information regarding the inception, development, anatomical configurations, and functions of the physical being and knowledge of the physical Earth, life, and the phenomena of the spiritual existence or spiritual consciousness.

Chiropractic has a spiritual component that is usually discussed when conversing in the philosophy of chiropractic. My impression is that the spiritual aspects of chiropractic are missing from most of the curriculums of chiropractic schools. It is interesting to note that spirituality in chiropractic has sometimes been shunned, while in the field of medicine, spirituality is currently being embraced.

Consider the work of neuroscientist Andrew Newberg, MD, Director of Research at Thomas Jefferson University Hospital. Dr. Newberg has published a series of twenty-four lectures called *The Spiritual Brain: Science and Religious Experience*. The lectures explore the new and exciting field of neuroethology, a discipline aimed at understanding the connections between our brains and religious phenomena. He uses an academic, experimental approach to prove that the nervous system is hard-wired for God.

The brain's neurophysiological structure and spirituality develop in parallel throughout a person's lifetime. Religious beliefs and practices have measurable, biological effects on the brain. The current neuroscientific data (via functional MRIs, EEGs, and SPECTS) help us to understand how God, religion, and spirituality are intertwined with ongoing nervous system development.

THE NEUROSKELETON

When D.D. Palmer discovered chiropractic, he discovered something that completely changed and rocked the world. The medical and scientific communities had unconscious and irrational reactions to the appearance of chiropractic on the scene; they responded with avoidance, denial, and a plan for extermination. This is a typical response to an overwhelming phenomenon that cannot be integrated in the ordinary way.

Palmer discovered that the creator of man designed the nervous system with a neuroskeleton. He found that the neuroskeleton can act as a tuner and regulator of the nervous system. His revelation was that the spinous and transverse processes of the twenty-four vertebrae in the vertebral column can serve as levers to fine-tune the nervous system, thereby allowing the energy of the nervous system to vibrate at a normal or even superior frequency. The vibrational frequency of the energy is the tone, which means that chiropractic revolves around tone.

Tone is the mean from which we measure the variations of organization, structure, temperature, flexibility, rigidity, tension, and elasticity. Quantum physics, quantum mechanics, energy, vibrational frequency, and tone are now the new paradigm of health; Palmer was talking this language in the 1880s.

In addition to utilizing the spinous and transverse processes as levers to fine-tune the nervous system, we can also use the cranial and facial bones to balance the tone of the nerve system. These bones make up the cranial facial neuroskeleton, as they house and protect the brain. It is important to realize that the skull is not one solid bone—it is made up of twenty-two individual bones that actually move every time we breathe—or at least, they are supposed to.

According to Dr. Marc Pick, Cranial Physiologist, every time we inhale, the ventricles of the brain collapse and produce cerebral spinal fluid, squeezing CSF out into the subdural space that surrounds the brain and the spinal cord. This causes an increased intrathecal pressure inside the cranium that must be accommodated for by a rhythmic expansion and relaxation of the cranium during respiration. To allow for this increased pressure, the skull expands every time we inhale. Every time we exhale, the skull relaxes and contracts.

Each of the cranial bones has their own specific direction of motion, which is imperative to normal cranial function and the function of the central nervous system. The primary bone of the cranial system is the sphenoid bone. It is the most centralized bone of the cranium and attaches the facial skeleton to the cranial vault. The sphenoid bone is often referred to as the "crucible bone," as it houses the pituitary gland, the "master gland" that controls the overall function of the endocrine system. This is important to understand, as normal sphenoid function and movement are an intricate part of normal pituitary function and overall endocrine function.

The main hinge of this dynamic, moveable cranial system is located at the sphenobasilar junction, where the occiput articulates with the sphenoid bone. This articulation is a symphasis joint, which is disc-like and allows for movement and the overall flexion and relaxation of the skull during respiration. Every time we inhale, the skull expands and the sphenobasilar junction goes into flexion. The occiput moves inferiorly and slightly anteriorly during this inhalation phase of respiration.

At the same time, the sacrum also moves in a similar fashion, with the sacral apex moving in a slightly anterior direction. This coordinated movement is facilitated by the dural attachment at the occiput and the sacrum, which acts like a lever between the two, forming the sacro-occipital pump. When the cranial system becomes fixated and its movements are impaired, the normal flow of cerebral spinal fluid throughout the brain and spinal cord is impeded, which alters the function of the nervous and endocrine systems, and directly affects normal body function. These cranial subluxations can be easily detected through testing procedures and corrected with the craniofacial technique as developed by chiropractor Dr. Adam Deltorto. CFR is based on SOT protocols which address aberrations at both the cranial and sacral ends of this CSF pumping mechanism clearing below the atlas before addressing the cranium.

Using brain imaging and other cutting-edge physiological studies, we now can understand how the brain controls or responds to religious and spiritual beliefs. For example, fMRI studies show that long-term practitioners of spiritual practices such as meditation have thicker and more active frontal lobes than those who don't.

The discoveries by our chiropractic forefathers revealed insights into human health that were once thought to be mystical. Presently, these principles are being discovered anew by our contemporaries in medicine and neuroscience. The principles of chiropractic are beyond quantum physics and reach into the world of quantum metaphysics. Quantum physics is the most efficient and proven scientific theory of all time.

Since chiropractic science comprises biology, the

science of vitalism, several PhDs and chiropractors are researching vitalism because it is essential for chiropractic. Chiropractic science acknowledges a spiritual existence in this world and the one to come. The doctrines of an afterlife are applicable in the liberation and movement toward vitalistic advancement.

Every year we see new techniques, imaging techniques, and ways of detecting and correcting vertebral subluxations. Scientists such as chiropractor and a neurophysiologist Heidi Haavik, PhD, are proving that correcting spinal dysfunction, or vertebral subluxations, improves brain function and restores tone to the nervous system. This is an area in chiropractic that needs to be studied diligently.

THE SPIRITUAL CHIROPRACTOR

In a typical medical treatment, physicians generally deal with the physical only, whereas chiropractors attenuate both the physical and the spiritual. The spirit holds the same relation to the body as God, the all-wise intelligence, does to the Universe. If you can locate the one, you can designate the location and define the limits of the other.

God is indwelling in the universe, everywhere present; He occupies every part thereof. Likewise, the spirit permeates every portion of the body in which it dwells. God does not depend on the universe for His existence, and neither does the spirit rely on the body for its continued manifestations.

The spiritual intelligence controls unintelligent matter through the nervous system. Each and every portion of the body is permeated by the spirit and its means of communication. The founder of chiropractic located the spirit in man, and found its abiding place to be throughout the entire body, a position from which each and every nerve ganglia may be used for receiving and forwarding impulses.

Education is as straightforward as it sounds. Each chiropractor has their personal area of expertise—the neuromusculoskeletal system—and the spiritualist has a general working knowledge of most spiritual paths. The spiritual chiropractor has the ability to reconnect the physical with the spiritual and understands the spiritual path. Here, the chiropractor acts as a spiritual guide until the client is able to access the inner guidance that enables them to take over for themselves.

D.D. Palmer's work is the backbone of the chiropractic philosophy. The practitioner meditates to daily renew, validate, and experience their own connection to God and teaches clients to do the same through a series of methods for exercising meditation skills.

Hundreds of studies show that religion has a measurable effect on health. For example, church attendance is associated with decreased heart disease, blood pressure, emphysema, cirrhosis, and suicide. Based on this cutting-edge scientific information, I suggest you consider spirituality as an integral tool in your mission of chiropractic.

UNIVERSAL INTELLIGENCE

As we know, any deviation from tone (the basis of chiropractic) is dis-ease. Now we need to concur that the philosophy of chiropractic deals with spirituality, a science of sciences, a science that explores the reality and properties of universal intelligence and our connection with it.

The potential of chiropractic is infinite when universal laws in regard to our physical and spiritual connection are scientifically comprehended. Are you ready to truly understand the chiropractic principles of spirit?

Chiropractic spirituality is mysteriously absent from today's chiropractic curriculum. The phrase "quantum spirit" is rarely spoken, even among chiropractic philosophers. There may be a few schools that delve into quantum physics, but not many teach the crown jewel of chiropractic philosophy, chiropractic quantum metaphysics.

Biology is not only the study of life but also a study of transcendent dimension, a realm beyond our physical earthly senses. John McAtamney, DC, wrote me a personal note on his perspective:

Universal intelligence has no solicitude. Universal intelligence is the thought of creation that God had that forms the universe. It is an aspect of God but does not define God. Universal intelligence is something we see expressed in matter. Since life expresses intelligence, it is universal life expressing itself through matter. It is the desire of God to live in his/her creation and have experiential knowledge available only when there is relationship between the creator and the created.

I am an eternal spirit expressing life through matter and that intelligence also includes an innate intelligence designed by the creator to handle the needs of daily life in my body from conception to death. Therefore, spirit can live fully in its relationship with its source. So, chiropractic connects man the physical with man the spiritual. We are an eternal spirit having a singular expression called life and have been imbued with the ability to live completely; mentally, physically, emotionally and spiritually.

The principles of chiropractic teach us about universal intelligence. The first principle, a theological principle, states, "Universal Intelligence is in all matter and continually gives to it all its properties and actions, thus maintaining it in existence." Palmer also wrote that chiropractic "is an educational, scientific, religious system. It associates its practice, belief and knowledge with that of religion. It imparts instruction relating both to this world and the world to come. Supreme spiritual existence can only be obtained through earthly experience."

According to research by Andrew Newberg, MD, in the field of neurology, Palmer was certainly on to something. Palmer went on to say that "man is dual entity, composed of intelligence and matter, spirit and material, the immortal and the mortal, the everlasting and the transient. . . . Chiropractors, especially, are aiding in this great advancement by adjusting the osseous structure, the position of which has to do with determining normal and abnormal tension . . . I hold it to be self-evident that all men and women who have acquired sufficient knowledge and skill to remove the nerve tension which prevents physical, mental and spiritual development, are engaged in a work of a higher order . . ."[1]

He went on to say, "I do not propose to change chiropractic . . . into a religion. The moral and religious duty of a chiropractor are not synonymous with the science, art and philosophy of chiropractic. There is a vast difference between a theological religion and a religious duty . . ." D.D. Palmer correlated the art of adjusting the neuroskeleton together with the philosophy of the science and art. Palmer's mission was—you guessed it—chiropractic.

MISSION CHIROPRACTIC

Palmer's son, B.J. Palmer, also found his mission in chiropractic, which can be seen by the long list of his literary works. B.J. wrote many brilliant and memorable statements. One passage of his work really hit home for me.

I have heard much about the Missionary schools—places where men are trained to save men's souls and bodies and keep them together—medical

---

[1] D.D. Palmer, *The Chiropractor*, 1914

missionaries—and we have reached the conclusion that a Chiropractic missionary training school would be fine. The Chiropractic missionary would not need paraphernalia with him (which in the other man's case were purchased with the pennies of perhaps thousands of confidence-abiding Sunday-schools, all confident that their pennies will convert and save the soul of some heathen). But what can you expect? When parents believe the way to save bodies is to poison them with vaccine virus, etc., how could you expect children to know better? It will take more of their money to transport these supplies and drug-store products to the other side—all this *would be saved*, and the Chiropractor could go about doing good free and untrammeled—tho he live in Africa. One year or forty, he is ready to restore normal conditions—he is not handicapped by lack of supplies or the wherewithal to overcome diseased conditions. If we were looking at this no more than from an economical or sociological standpoint it is worthwhile. I will, someday, establish a Palmer Missionary Institute in Davenport and start out missionaries.[2]

---

2 B.J. Palmer, *The Philosophy and Principles of Chiropractic Adjustments*, 1911

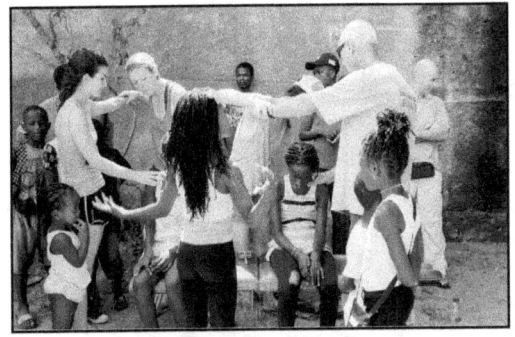

Brian Long, DC and Becky Long, DC channeling energy.

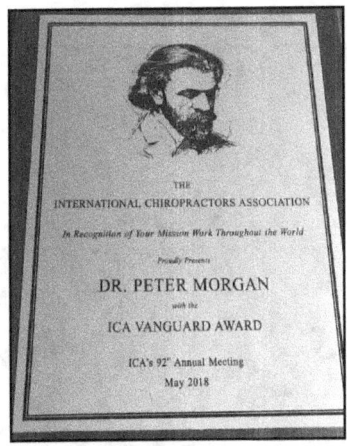

This award was given to me right around my 92nd mission trip.

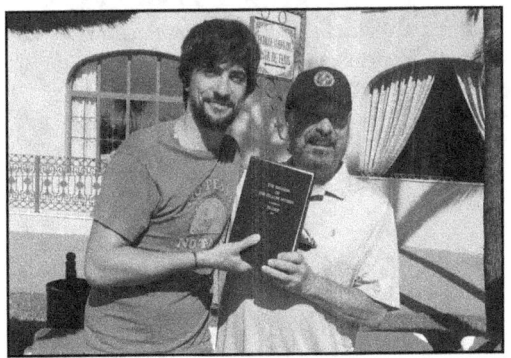

Sebastian Fuentes, DC and I at chiroeurope
celebrating the bigness of the fellow within!

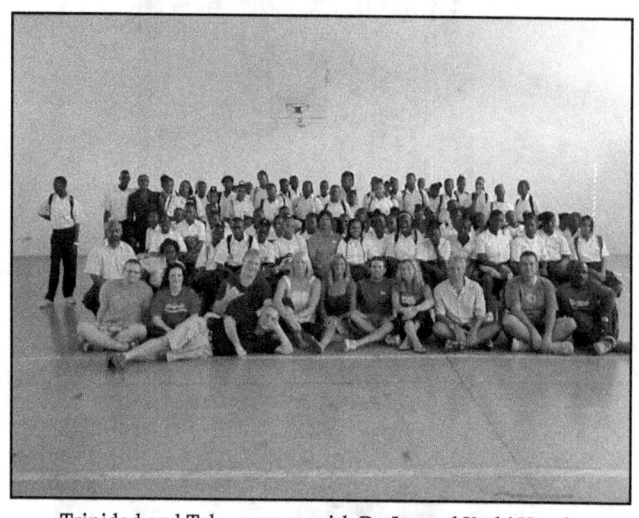

Trinidad and Tobago 2009 with Dr. Jay and Kathi Handt.

CHAPTER 2

Chiropractic Humanitarians

*We make a living by what we get,
but we make a life by what we give.*

—WINSTON CHURCHILL

A major focus that I have is to promote chiropractic humanitarianism around the world, which raises the question, what is a chiropractic humanitarian? The ways in which we all help others, from the patients we see daily in our offices to the world's poorest children we meet on missions makes us all humanitarians.

As chiropractic humanitarians, we believe that improving human welfare is a moral imperative and that by correcting vertebral subluxations we help to alleviate the suffering of others. Chiropractic humanitarians strive to ensure that those who are poor or who have suffered traumatic events receive a chiropractic adjustment so that they can cope with the physical, mental, and emotional stress they are called on to endure.

Chiropractic humanitarians are strong professionals, students, and lay people. They are male and female; young and old; and of all colors, cultures, ideologies, and backgrounds. Their motivations for humanitarian work are diverse, but they are all united by their commitment to humanitarianism and chiropractic. Chiropractic humanitarians strive to provide assistance to the increasing number of people affected by manmade and natural disasters every year. They reach out to the poorest and neediest people regardless of where they are in the world or what nationality, social, or religious group they belong to. They reflect everything that is good and compassionate about our profession and our humanity, and they should be respected and supported financially.

We face a future in which more humanitarian aid will be needed. If chiropractic humanitarians do not have full access to those in need, many thousands of people will not receive the chiropractic care they require. The best way to ensure chiropractic humanitarians can fulfill their mission is by improving awareness of and respect for the principles on which chiropractic work is conducted.

In theory, humanitarian work is simple: you help people in need. But knowing how to help others is not always easy. The World Chiropractic Alliance, in its role as a non-governmental organization affiliated with the United Nations Department of Public Information, is in a unique position to support and publicize a variety of chiropractic missions. This is why it is so important to support the efforts of chiropractic humanitarians everywhere.

A MISSION CHIROPRACTOR'S STORY

Many missionaries have submitted writings of their experiences in Haiti and Dominican Republic after they returned from one of Mission International's mission trips, and everyone has a different impression of the poorest nation in the western hemisphere. In 2010, Haiti suffered a catastrophic earthquake that killed more than 220,000 people and injured even more. The following story was written by Joseph Cucci, DC, who attended one of our mission trips two months after the earthquake in Haiti in 2010. An edited version is reprinted here with permission.

Haiti. Its name reveals the nature of a nation: Hades, as in Zeus's evil brother. Hell on Earth. After the earthquake, there was no such thing as a shower or running water that I could see. It hit me like a wave that 3 million people hadn't had a shower since the earthquake two months before. Dozens of children without clothes defecated on the side of the road, with no way to clean themselves or the street.

The sides of roads were piled high with garbage, like mounds of snow after a storm. Sitting on top of the garbage were people selling foods of all kinds. They made little charcoal fires to cook animal organs and corn, handling everything with filthy hands. Lying on the sides of the street were dozens of dead dogs, cats, and chickens. A horse stood with its intestines hanging out of its abdomen.

We slept at the house of one of Dr. Peter Morgan's patients, a famous Haitian comedian named Boss Massel. Everyone in Haiti knows him, even though he now drives a taxi in New York City. He sends money to his wife and a community of children he houses and feeds.

There were many, many children living in tents on the property adjacent to Boss's house, which he also owns. Some of the other mission members brought tents donated by the Lions Club.

On the night we arrived, I was exhausted from the drive and overwhelmed by the situation. I went to bed at eight o'clock. My sleeping bag gave me no comfort as I lay on the concrete roof of Boss's house, where many of the volunteers were sleeping. As I lay there, I wondered if I had gotten myself in over my head on this chiropractic mission.

The morning came, and I had not slept a wink. To my surprise, however, I was full of energy and ready to give the unique and vital gift of chiropractic. I looked over the side of the roof and saw coal burning on an open fire and a pot propped up to boil water. Next to the pot stood an orphan girl washing dishes; the dishwater was brown, and she was scrubbing the dishes with her bare hands. She had was stacking the still-dirty plates and silverware on a muddy cinder block.

I looked over the back side of the roof and saw a boy standing in a pile of burnt garbage, squatting and defecating. I would find out later that this town had some of the cleanest conditions in Haiti.

Boss's wife, Shirley, was a good woman with a kind face, but she was very pushy. I could not fault her for it. I guess any woman caring for and housing hundreds of orphans would be pushy. It seemed half my energy was spent resisting her as she persistently said, "Eat, eat." I finally had to tell her, "American stomachs are weak and cannot handle many things." After seeing the plates and silverware being washed, I would rather eat off the floor of my car with a stick from a tree than use one of those utensils.

Peter partook of everything. He drank the coffee and ate the food like he was at a five-star hotel. Breakfast was coffee, spaghetti with ketchup, and a bottle of ketchup on the side if you wanted more. We were served spaghetti and ketchup for breakfast every morning.

After breakfast, Dr. Morgan went with Boss and an array of people from Haiti who did political work with the government to try to establish the legal work necessary for the orphanage, a chiropractic center, and an educational center in Haiti.

As my team and I drove through Port au Prince, we saw that the devastation was outrageous. People were sitting on top of the houses, churches, and government buildings, which had all been reduced to rubble. The National Palace, a government building similar in function to the White House in the United States, had crumbled to the ground and was in shambles. There was destruction everywhere.

The first place we stopped was a tent city. There were hundreds if not thousands of tent cities made up of families living on top of each other. The "tents" were made of clothes propped up by sticks. We went to a community that Mission Life International had adopted through a bishop and his wife.

Dr. Morgan had been to Haiti five times in the two months since the earthquake. The people knew him and knew why we were there. When we got out of the car, we were immediately surrounded by thousands of people. A local man named Eddie, the only Haitian I met who could speak English, was acting as our guide and bodyguard. We tried to have Eddie tell everyone to get into lines, but the sheer mass of people made it impossible.

We had three tables and three chiropractors. Between us, we adjusted hundreds of people in two hours. That sounds impossible, but the boundary of what is possible gets lost when there is so great a need. We adjusted subluxated specific by innate guidance. It took seconds for us to adjust the thoracic and the cervical spine or neck. Before the first person was off the table, the second was getting on.

As you lose yourself in service, the educated mind takes a back seat. The innate mind takes over, and that is when miracles happen. I saw people having to be lifted onto a table be able to walk off. I saw crossed eyes straighten. Countless masses received more life and more connection between body and mind and man to God.

One of our volunteers was overwhelmed as she dressed wounds, open sores that had not been treated since the quake. Malaria was prevalent, and fevers ran high. All of these people had a greater chance of survival after an adjustment than they had before.

Eddie kept us somewhat safe and taught us that different tent villages had different personalities. Some were extremely dangerous, like the tent village in front of the collapsed National Palace, and some were hospitable, even gracious, like the bishop's and Mission Life's tent villages.

We went to a hospital for children, where most of the patients were amputees. Many suffered from nerve and other diseases of all kinds. The head doctor, an Irish woman who had lived in Haiti for ten years, was excited to see us. One medical doctor told me about the miraculous changes that had taken place with many of the children after they are adjusted by our earlier mission chiropractic groups. She introduced me to a child whose face used to be sunken in and had returned to normal after an adjustment. Chiropractic is most noticeable in children's diseases because childhood is when the most innate life force permeates the body. This helps their ability to grow and form cells and tissues in the body.

The emotional anguish was heart-wrenching. Though we were on a mission of healing, love, and kindness, there was still tension within our group, as none of us knew how to deal with the overwhelming situation, and we all had low blood sugar and dehydration. We ate and drank water, but the diet was poor and there was not enough drinking water. It was so hot that at times I felt like I would pass out.

The mind, however, is the most powerful thing any man knows. Through concentration and commitment, we find we can endure more than we think. By the second night I found myself so weak that I ate the rice and beans Shirley that served for dinner. As I was eating, I thought it better to die with these children we were feeding than to die alone on the streets of Haiti. From that night on, I ate with the three hundred or so children whom Mission Life had brought food to from the money we raised. The children were happy. Every night we sang songs, danced, and played games together. I found endless amounts of love in their eyes.

Dr. Morgan started an orphanage in days with the help of Boss's star power in the country and the pastor of the community church. I was unsure if it was my purpose to help start an orphanage. I have always been a chiropractic purist, but with this new orphanage, these children would get ongoing chiropractic care. With further funding, we could build a chiropractic center and an educational center, so I signed papers and received an official government card granting me the authority to legally adopt homeless children from outside of the country. After seeing the suffering of these children, I could only accept what innate had provided.

That Thursday I was informed that my spiritual father and chiropractic mentor, Pasqaule Cerasoli, died at the age of ninety-nine on March 1, 2010. I cried. Of course, I knew from his teaching that these were selfish tears. Pasquale once said, "Why is it so easy to find the beauty of dying leaves but not in dying people?"

That night I was asked to speak at the community church. I spoke Pasquale's message of love. That night I found comfort in the children's song and dance and in the knowing that in his passing we are closer now than we could be in the physical life.

I was full of energy when the sun came up. Knowing it was our last day, I wanted to leave everything on the field. We had fed many children; brought clothes; and provided shelter, glasses, toothpaste, and water, but this was my last day to serve chiropractically. Our team worked harder on that day than on any other. Going from tent city to tent city, we were constantly adjusting.

Through the laying on of hands, the loving and caring for the patients, the belief, the healing that took place in this one day, I easily gave more adjustments than I had for the entire year, and likely more than in two years in practice. Every single patient I touched came off my table with a smile and gratitude in their heart.

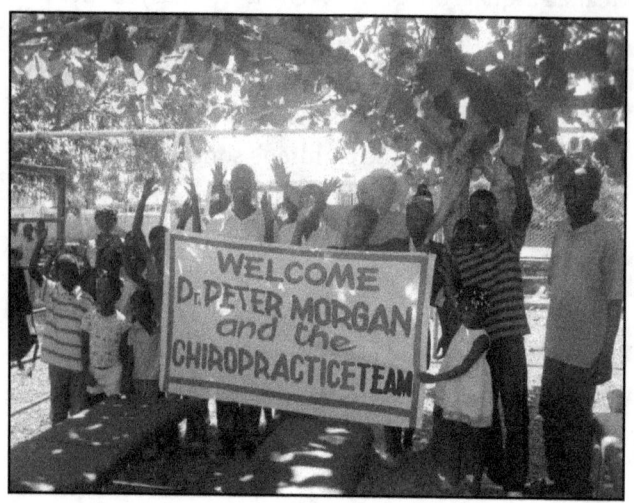

A nice welcome to Ft. Liberte, Haiti. 2008

CHAPTER 3

Mission Chiropractic

"Mission," from the Latin missum:
A specific task that a person or group has been
charged with or adopts as their main purpose.

Chiropractic is the healing tool of chiropractic missionaries. A chiropractic adjustment is a tool from the chiropractic missionary to the patient for the purpose of reconnecting the physical with the spiritual.

The term "chiropractic missionary" is used here to describe the personal commitment of an individual to the opening of the world to the concepts of drugless healing. Not all chiropractic missionaries are chiropractors. There are chiropractic missionaries from all walks of life, all areas of human endeavor, and they focus the concepts of drugless healing and helping the poor through their own particular perspective.

Chiropractors who go on chiropractic missions encounter a remarkable and wondrous journey filled with love and compassion. This genuine love is bestowed upon humankind, especially the poor and needy. These missions are to alleviate the suffering of others, especially the poor. The universe plans something special for every chiropractic mission, and we can make a difference by administering chiropractic and help with the change of the world.

Any one of us can change the course of humanity. One individual can affect millions of people. Our calling is to save lives. We are instruments of the universe and are asked to enlighten others about chiropractic. We have been chosen to give something back.

PRAYER FOR CELEBRATION OF CHIROPRACTIC

Today we come to celebrate our call, to celebrate our gifts, and to remember how much the world needs us. Through blessing our hands, we acknowledge that they are holy hands, given to fulfill divine purposes. This blessing symbolizes our belief in the sacredness of our everyday lives and the sacred work we do with our hands. Through this blessing, we recognize the divine presence with us here and now.

Spirit of wisdom, we come seeking You for the work of healing You have given our hands to do. Thank You for working through our hands to provide healing. We thank You for the privilege of using our hands to those in pain and suffering for Your healing. You have given us special hands to touch one another's lives with comfort and healing. May we use our gifts to bring healing to those whom You place in our care. Bless our hearts and hands, Holy wisdom, and guide us to use them to make whole what is broken in our world.

CHIROPRACTORS AND OUR FUTURE

Do you ever wonder about the future of chiropractic? Have you heard the question, "If you were the last chiropractor on the planet, would chiropractic survive?" I am here to tell you that chiropractic is in great hands. Chiropractic is safe.

We sometimes have chiropractic students come on our mission trips, and they are truly on a mission to serve humanity with compassion and love. I am honored to serve with these young chiropractors, and I learn many valuable lessons from them.

After one mission trip in particular, the students conveyed a message to the chiropractic community:

We are the future of chiropractic, and chiropractic is in good hands. We are determined, dedicated, powerful and passionate. We are determined to create a world where every man, woman, and child are under chiropractic care, a world where each individual is mentally, physically, and chemically in tune with the innate that animates life.

We have dedicated our lives to protecting the sacred principles of chiropractic, to make sure that the masses are educated and fully understand its importance.

We know what is going on in the world today, we know what needs to be done, and we know that we have the power within ourselves to make it happen. Our passion for chiropractic will attract every person who comes into contact with us. We are the future. We are chiropractic.

The common thread in all chiropractic practices is that chiropractors value every human being as being fully connected to or is a manifestation of God. Each chiropractor experiences that connection in their lifework, and encourages others to experience their own connection, thus leading to developing their own lifework goals.

In the future, movie and television writers, musicians, artists, and even the commercial ads will be working with Chiromission themes. Science scholars and philosophers, too, have their representatives. Much of the work on quantum physics is developed through the chiropractic perspectives, as is the growing acceptance of alternative health care methods in the general community.

New understandings in health, life, creativity, art, philosophy, spiritualism, psychology, and sociology all have taken D.D. Palmer's concepts and restructured them within the framework of New Age views. Palmer was ahead of his time. It is important to read his works to get a detailed description of innate and God.

Perhaps by now you have make the shift in your thought process. Your intentions are on service—serving humankind with love and compassion. By embarking on mission chiropractic, you are beginning a remarkable and wondrous journey, and you will encounter riches beyond your wildest dreams.

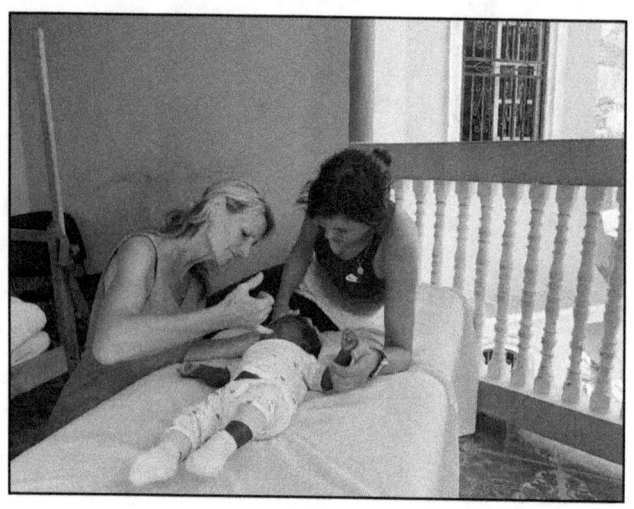

Drs. Mary Ellen Stephens and Emmie Van Niekerk
are incredible missionaries.

CHAPTER 4

Innate Intelligence

*I have found that among its other benefits,
giving liberates the soul.*

—MAYA ANGELOU

In personal practice, the chiropractor realizes that the connection to God is found within each living entity; therefore, each person is capable of becoming conscious of that connection and living in accordance with it. The chiropractor understands that there is an innate intelligence that runs the body.

An understanding of the individual spirituality is of utmost importance. The implication is that each person has a divine purpose directed by God as well as an individual purpose directed by innate intelligence. Most of the time, these two purposes can seem to be in opposition. I contend that they are meant to work together, to exist together in harmony, and to complement each other. I contend that through readings of the Bible the dualistic purpose will be known, and as you become aware and ascend into the higher dimension of your life, these two purposes will no longer be dualistic. You will have achieved something very special.

Spiritual growth through compassion and love service gives you the tools to make your everyday life work and to bring increasingly higher levels of order, harmony, clarity, and love into every area of your life. You will begin to see the true purpose and mission of your life. As you link your mind with God, you will gain more awareness of the path of human evolution and your part in it. You will attract the tools to carry out your mission in life.

Your life's mission can affect the whole world. You can be a leader of this movement and help create more harmony in our world. You can affect the animal and plant kingdom, as well. You will be able to do what you always wanted to do. You will love what you do, and you will want to do it all the time.

SPIRITUAL GROWTH

As you begin your spiritual growth and let love and compassion into your life, you will ascend to higher dimensions of your life. You will see the world differently. As you become more aware and grow spiritually, you will begin to communicate differently. You will attract loving relationships and connect with people in higher ways. You will begin to share more and ascend to higher levels of intimacy. You will have an incredible connection with your family and be able to connect with others in a meaningful and loving way.

One of the first things you can do to grow spiritually is to let go of any preconceived notions that you have about spiritual growth. Spiritual growth occurs when you attempt to help humanity, just as Jesus did. It occurs when you raise the consciousness of service, compassion, and love you provide to humanity. Spiritual growth also occurs as you connect with your higher self, or your innate intelligence. Your innate intelligence is coalesced with God, and God will send you messages in the form of intuition and feelings, such as hunches. Go with these feelings.

You are blessed because you have a special purpose, a special function, and a special mission, and they will give your life a very spiritual dimension—the ability for your innate intelligence to connect with your soul. As you communicate with your innate intelligence and let it work without hindrance, you connect with your soul. You will start to notice odd things happening. You will attract loving things and money into your life. This money will help you with your mission of serving humanity. People, newspapers, radio, and television will bring you messages from God. Your spiritual growth will increase tremendously as you become aware of your innate intelligence.

CONNECTING WITH YOUR INNATE INTELLIGENCE

If you have trouble connecting with your innate intelligence, try imagining that you have a wise teacher or advisor who lives with you all the time and has a direct line of communication with Jesus. Visualize this wise old teacher speaking with you daily, coaching and advising you on matters of importance. This teacher advises you on how you can bring more love and compassion to the world and how you can help people in impoverished nations or in your own community. Listen to your wise old teacher on matters of finance, love, spirituality, and personal relationships.

After you have practiced these visualizations and communications for one month, you can stop imagining, because you will be connected with your innate intelligence. (My innate intelligence is advising me at this moment on what words I should write on this paper.) As you get more in tune with your innate intelligence, allow it to become the director of every part of your life. Once you connect with your innate intelligence on a daily basis, you will seek to learn, experience, create, compose, write, and paint. You will seek to illuminate, speak, run, climb, jump, help, serve, and explore the greater being that you are. You will uncover the mysteries of God, and you will never be the same.

Your innate intelligence also runs your physical body. As long as the innate intelligence is allowed to connect to every cell in your body, your body will be healthy. Your soul is your spiritual connection to God. God runs all the dimensions, all the galaxies, all of the unexplained phenomenon. The connection between the innate intelligence and God is profound. Man is not divisible. We are physical and spiritual. For physical growth we run, jump, lift weights, and so on. For spiritual growth, we need to strive to help humanity.

After you experience the joy of providing the service of compassion and love to humankind, you will never again want to slow down or stop. I feel like hugging the whole world. I cannot get enough hugs.

From time to time, your wise old teacher will give you tasks. You see, we all have a purpose for being on this Earth. God will unveil your mission and purpose as you serve. God planned something very special for you, and He requests that you make a difference. You are to minister and facilitate the change of the world. One person can change the course of humanity. It can be any one of us. One individual can affect millions of others.

Since you are reading these passages, you are one of the chosen few to perform this work. Your calling is to save lives. You are now an instrument of God. You are requested to enlighten others. You were chosen to give something back. Think about what you have already received: You can read. You can see. You have wealth beyond your wildest dreams. Now it is time to give back. It is time to serve. You were created for a life of good deeds. As you perform these assignments, you will be fulfilling your life's purpose.

You have been entrusted with a special mission, a sacred oath. Listen carefully to your wise old teacher, your innate intelligence, to give you your unique and special task. Your teacher has been consulting with Jesus. When you fulfill this endeavor, the rewards will be the greatest treasures of them all: love, serenity, and joy.

Material wealth will probably accompany, as well; however, this is not why we serve. Material wealth cannot be the focus of service. We serve because we have been chosen by God, and God will reward us. We may not know when or how, but it will happen.

There is an abundance of everything in the universe; there is a lack of nothing. It is better to give and not think of receiving. World-renowned speaker, motivational coach, and author Bob Proctor said that learning to truly give without thought of receiving is the best way to learn to trust abundance. Each time you give, think to yourself, "There's plenty to go around." This is why service is such an important element of our purpose. Focus on service, and abundance will come. When we serve for the sake of service, we open up our hearts to receive. This is the natural law of giving and receiving.

A piano or a violin can exist for centuries. Over time, the wood decays, yet if the instrument is in tune, it can sing sweet songs. The same thing occurs in living organisms. Our lives are energy, and they vibrate at a certain frequency. If your body is in proper tune, it will vibrate at a higher frequency. The vibrations can attract wonderful things into your life. When you are in tune, your vibrations are in tune with nature. You can actually see a healthy person in tune with the universe.

Think about the relationship you have with your soul. Your world is a reflection of that relationship. When things are working right, your physical body is vibrating with a harmonious frequency. You are in tune with nature; you are vibrating with nature, in tune with your spirit. Your spirit is the highest vibrational "you"—the embodiment of your spirit—and your interface between human and divine.

Your innate intelligence runs your physical body but also gives insight to your relationship with the physical world. Innate helps you to attract into your life the things that you think about. Your soul is the connection between the innate intelligence and the universal intelligence. Spirit is the combination of the innate intelligence, the soul, and the universal intelligence.

When the body dies, innate intelligence and the soul evolve into a higher spiritual plane and leave the body. The vibratory frequency and tone change, and a "growth spurt" occurs. The spirit continually evolves, with slight vibratory changes. It will eventually coalesce and vibrate at the same frequency as universal intelligence and become one with it. Before that time, the spirit will be one with universal intelligence yet vibrate at a different frequency. Many times additional growth is necessary, and the process will need to duplicate but at a higher plane. This is often termed a rebirth or reincarnation.

PRAYER FOR UNIVERSAL BRILLIANCE

Oh, great universe, pass your healing light into our spiritual consciousness, down, down into our brain, our physical consciousness, the seat of our soul. Down, down into our cords, then along our nerves, and through our hands so that we may serve our brothers and sisters throughout the world who live and die in poverty and hunger. Through our hands, give them the unaltered nervous system, thereby creating energy and restoring tone, so they can enjoy life in this world and the one to come.

Oh, great universe, pass us the knowledge and skill to remove nerve tension, which prevents physical, mental, and spiritual development. Give us the power of love so we can create peace and joy.

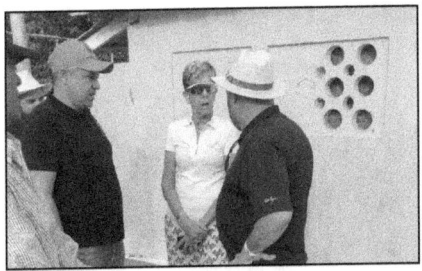

Fidelio Sanchez has been the Mission Life International Director of the Dominican Republic for over ten years.

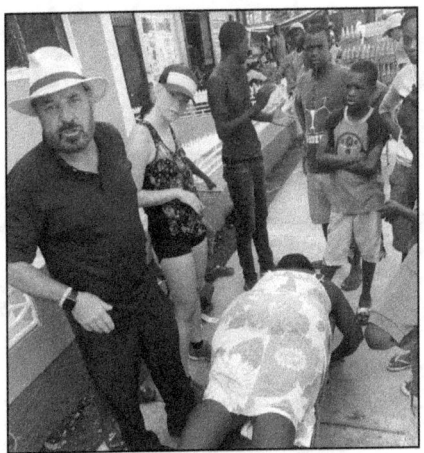

In Haiti we are called the "Touch Healers"

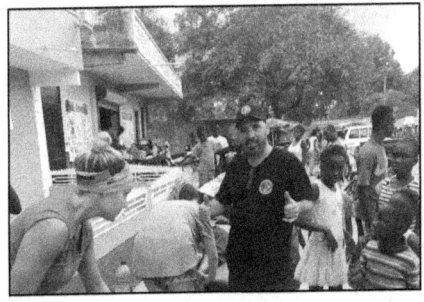

In front of Alex Thoni's cousins grocery store. Ouanaminthe, Haiti.

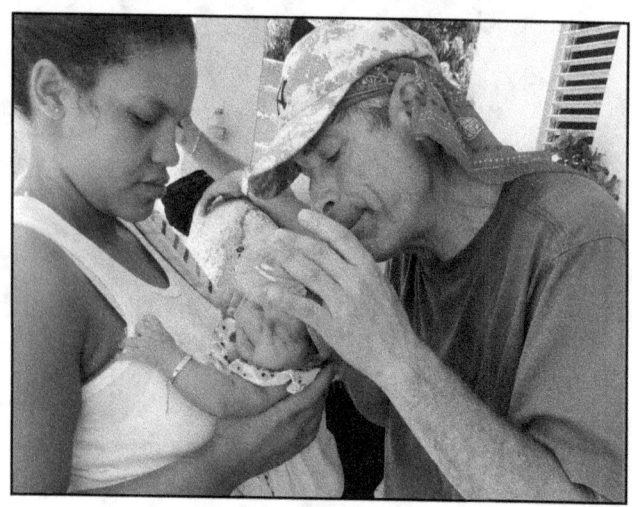

Dr. Henri Rosenblum has healing hands.

CHAPTER 5

Joy and Serenity through Service

If we could change ourselves, the tendencies in the world would also change. As a man changes his own nature, so does the attitude of the world change towards him. . . .
We need not wait to see what others do.

—MOHANDAS GANDHI

Being a servant requires making a shift in our thought process. It is an inspirational adjustment to a noble manifestation. Our intention must be simply serving. Our purpose is to serve with love in our hearts. This alone will create something magnificent.

We begin by aiding people—assisting the poor and disabled, serving at homeless shelters, feeding the hungry at soup kitchens, and volunteering in missions to impoverished countries. We serve with love and compassion, excitement and joy. It is such an uplifting endeavor. It is an act of giving of ourselves without wanting anything in return, serving for the sake of serving.

This is the birth of an outstanding spiritual voyage. An outward journey is important, fantastic, and lots of fun; however, the heart-centered inner journey brings light to our spiritual self, our mission, and our purpose. As servants, we think more about others than ourselves. We focus on others; we forget about ourselves and think only of others. We lose ourselves in service, and wonderful transformations result.

Through service we encounter a remarkable and wondrous expedition. We experience flourishing careers, wonderful families, abundant material goods, financial security, respected roles in our professions. We become spiritual leaders in our community. It is incredible, a magnificent journey. These are the blessings that are waiting for you.

REQUIREMENTS FOR SERVICE

A mission, purpose, and intention to serve is the foundation of mission chiropractic. Empathy and sincerity are essential. Love and kindness are prerequisites. You will bestow love and benevolence upon people, especially the poor, the hungry, the destitute, and those of impoverished countries. You will serve to relieve those who are suffering, the stressed and the destitute. You will serve with love.

Love is the gift that was passed on to us through God. Service is the noble virtue that passes on love from man to man. It is a natural law. It is this virtue that unifies us and inspires our lives. The great artists, architects, and poets were blessed with this divine virtue. The people of underdeveloped and developing nations certainly need this service. Our communities need this service.

Genuine love and compassion are demanding requirements. They require the transformation of self. Servants think more about others than themselves.

THE WINDOW WASHER

Years ago in New York City, there were countless car window washers on the streets. I didn't like them and always tried to avoid them. I would put my windshield wipers on whenever they approached my car. I would spray the fluid and move my car up so they would approach the car behind me instead. I don't see that many window washers now, but I see lots of them when I am in developing countries.

One day in the summer of 2012, when I was in a mission in Dominican Republic, I was picking up some missionaries from a church. I had just gotten off with the phone with my son. He had just passed his driver's test and was so happy. As our call ended, I was approached by a sixteen-year-old Haitian boy, the same age as my son.

He said to me, "Do you mind if I tell you my life's mission?" "No," I replied. He stuttered as he continued. "I am taking care of my brother, who is five years old, and my three-year-old sister. My parents died recently in an accident. My siblings and I are illegal here in Dominican Republic, and even though we have never been in Haiti, we can be deported there at any time. My mission is to get money to support my brother and sister."

This young man's name was Angel. He invited me to visit where he and his siblings lived. We walked along grimy, mud-covered pathways, and when we arrived to their aluminum shack, I saw that it was among hundreds of other shacks and mud huts. Angel's shack had mucky dirt floors and a sheet hung up to separate clothes and other items dumped in a heap from the rest of the shack.

I asked Angel where he got the money to pay for the place. I figured it cost ten dollars a month. He answered, "I am a window washer." We were among hundreds of shacks, and there were no windows anywhere in sight. I asked, "Where do you wash windows?" He said, "I go up to the highway each day and wash the windows on the cars at the red lights."

I now love window washers. Whenever I see any window washers, I pull up close to make sure I get my windows cleaned even if they are spotless.

Angel eventually became a translator on our mission trips.

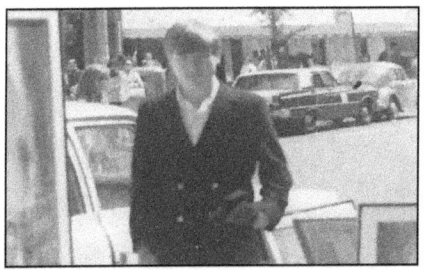

Selling Artwork in NYC in 1969. The next week I went to Woodstock and worked in a medical tent for 4 days helping people who were suffering from taking too much LSD.

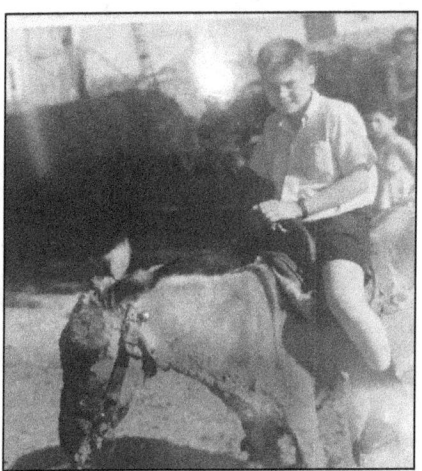

Thinking about doing a mission trip way back in 1965.

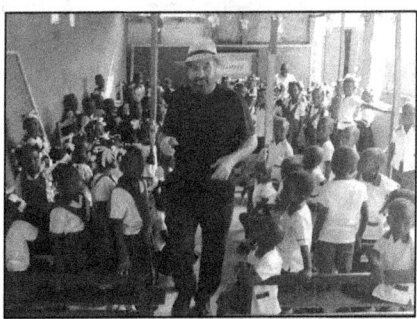

I love visiting our children's school in Ouanaminthe, Haiti.

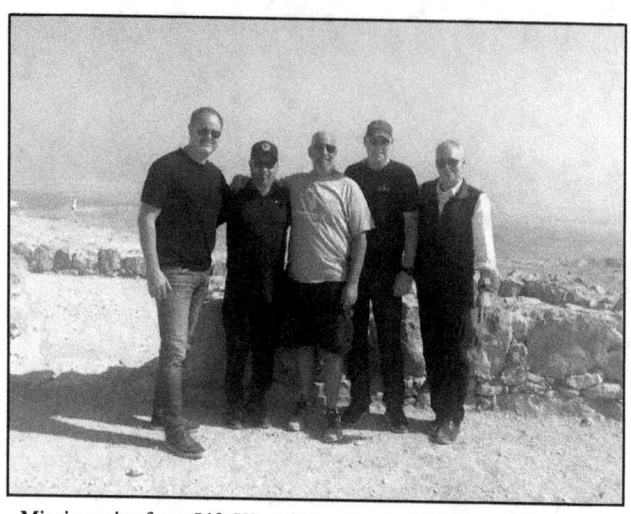
Missionaries from Life West Chiropractic College and I in Israel.

CHAPTER 6

Your Chiropractic Mission

My religion is very simple. My religion is kindness.
—THE DALAI LAMA

Each of us has a service to provide, and every service is important. There is no such thing as a small service; every service is desperately needed, and every service matters to the universe. The service that you give will come from your talents, your excitement, and your gifts. As you serve, more talents will become available to you. You will learn to draw, paint, and write through your passion to serve.

Energy will flow into your life, to and through you. You will feel a wave motion go through your body. One of the things I teach is how to connect with the wave motion that occurs in your body. This wave motion clears out the stress in your body and readjusts your spine. Have you ever watched a cat stretch its spine? The wave will take you through this same series of stretches. It will come as you serve humanity.

This increase in energy comes as you go through your spiritual growth. Every thought of humanity service you have, every emotion, initiates energy, which travels along waves across the universe. These waves, similar to radio waves, reach others with the same thought patterns and attract them to your purpose. Once these waves are flowing through you, you will encounter people ready to help you in your service. You will bring into alignment people with similar visions and immediately help the world move toward a better place.

Once you undertake your journey as a chiropractic missionary, you will receive love and compassion. The journey will enable you to go from anger, anxiety, and frustration to serenity and joy. Most importantly, you will discover your mission in life and discover God's purpose for your life.

PRAYER FOR A CALLING

God, you have called us here to affirm the dedication of our lives to chiropractic. We are your hands. You have blessed us with your healing power. God, we are comforted by the assurance of your constant presence at our side and of Your healing energy in our hands. Continue to bless our hands and the sacred work that they do.

Let our hands bring us joy, connection, and meaning. May our hands be sensitive, feeling what words cannot say. May they be tender, bringing loving witness to suffering. May they be strong and useful, bringing into the world what is needed. May they channel light and express the love in the divine heart.

Thank you, God, for the power you have put in our hands so that they will bring healing to all the people we touch. We are truly changing the world by touching lives. Thank you for this wonderful and most sacred blessing of our healing hands.

MISSION TRIP TO DOMINICAN REPUBLIC, 2006

I would like to tell you about one of our mission trips to Dominican Republic. On September 28, 2006, we arrived in Puerto Plata, Dominican Republic, on a spiritual mission. Our team comprised chiropractors Todd Herald, JC Doornick, Doreen Sundin, Craig Fishell, Marti and Dave Hecht, and me. Our purpose was to promote chiropractic and adjust all those who were subluxated throughout the world, especially in underprivileged countries, where resources are so terribly limited. We also wanted to cultivate students of chiropractic from those deprived areas so they could return to their beloved countries and work as chiropractors.

Shortly after our arrival, Todd, JC, and I were interviewed on two different television stations. During the interviews, we announced that chiropractic would be available in five locations over the following two days.

The next day we went to a local church, where

hundreds of people were waiting to be adjusted by our seven-chiropractor team. Some of them had been waiting since five o'clock that morning. People showed up with their children and great-grandparents, all wanting to receive God's greatest gift to man—chiropractic. More than two thousand people came to the church over the course of the day.

Partway through the day, some of the team went to orphanages. The children at these orphanages were severely disabled and had been abandoned in the streets. They all were adjusted that day. When I met up with Todd and JC during dinner, they looked tired and sad. Todd had to leave dinner early, and vomited for three hours. Apparently, he had to purge his sadness.

The next morning, we were up at five o'clock and ready to go. It was Saturday, September 30, 2006, a date I will never forget. We were split up and sent to three different locations. JC and I teamed up with two nuns, a medical director from a remote hospital, and an assistant. The six of us drove in a small four-passenger vehicle. One of the overweight nuns took turns sitting on JC's and my laps. We drove for two hours through the jungle mountains without air conditioning.

It was at least 100 degrees. We arrived at a small city at eight o'clock. People were arriving on the backs of mules to see us. We adjusted about two hundred people by ten thirty when I witnessed my first miracle.

People suddenly started yelling and screaming. They ran up to me, pointing, and urged me to run toward the street. A man who had just exited the hospital had collapsed and was apparently dying. JC ran over to him and found that the man had no pulse. JC adjusted the man's atlas, and immediately the man opened his eyes and motioned with his arms, as if a wave of energy were going through him. I gave the fellow some water, and he gradually came to his feet. Twenty-five people witnessed this, and our Dominican assistant captured it on video.

We went back to our post and adjusted every priest in the parish. We were then invited to eat at one of the priest's home. We had a very tasty lunch, although I was not familiar with any of the foods.

After lunch, we drove about another hour to a hospital in a small, mountainous city. Hundreds of people were waiting outside the hospital to be adjusted. JC and I were first given a tour of the hospital, and then we adjusted every doctor, every nurse, and every patient there. When we were done, the doors were opened for the people waiting outside. I adjusted twenty-two people in the first hour.

I slowed down considerably during the next several hours. JC and I adjusted people from newborn to well over a hundred. Most adjustments were to the upper cervical, and I felt I was an instrument of the universe. Even though I adjusted twenty-two people in one hour, I am confident that each patient received the perfect adjustment. It was as if time had slowed.

As we worked, our assistants were tasked with

telling waiting patients the chiropractic story: Chiropractic reunites the physical with the spiritual. The chiropractor releases the wisdom of the doctor within.

Night was approaching, and we had to take the long, winding drive back to our base. All I could think of was how happy and appreciative the people were to receive chiropractic. Strangely, I felt that I had received the greatest chiropractic gift that day.

When Todd and I met up that night, he shared another chiropractic miracle with me. One of the young patients at the orphanage was listless and had not moved or talked the day before. Todd told me that the boy was three and a half years old and unable to walk. He was examined for subluxations, and during the adjustment, the boy started crying very loudly and was very frightened. When Todd and Dave went to the orphanage three days later, the boy was running around and started urging Todd and Dave to adjust everyone in the orphanage.

These are just some of the stories we brought back with us after a wonderful time of sharing and caring for people who would not have had the benefits and healing of chiropractic any other way. During our four days in DR, we adjusted people in schools, churches, and orphanages. It was a truly rewarding experience.

Dr. Doreen Sundin said, "It was awesome to adjust people at a pace I didn't think was humanly possible and then have them come back the next day looking for me with a big smile on their face to tell me they felt 'mucho mejor' (much better). It was beyond awesome. All of those things and much more made this a memorable experience, but what will always be etched in my mind is the overwhelming sense of inner strength I personally walked away with, knowing that I had made a difference."

Dr. Marti Hecht said, "I was not sure what to expect when I first found out what my role was to be, but I have to say that the people of the DR were so warm and welcoming. The many patients we saw were there because they knew we could make a difference in their lives. Many came from miles away with the hope of feeling better, and they left knowing that we helped them. All day long we received thanks and smiles from each patient even if we could not communicate by words.

"One moment that stands out occurred while Dave and I were at a small church about forty-five minutes from town. We were in a small room with two windows, and had six chairs to see people. At one point, I looked outside, and there at least fifteen children of all ages peering in through one of the windows with such curiosity. The next thing we know, the whole room was filled with children—those who were looking in, then more and more. Some left to bring back their siblings. They all left with huge smiles. It was great to be appreciated. It was a tremendous feeling to be able to give, just to give. It definitely made me hope that our own patients could be so grateful."

Dr. Dave Hecht expressed his feelings about the

mission trip. "I am walking on a cloud. To be able to affect so many people in such a short amount of time was incredible. To be able to deliver the goods with minimal verbal communication and know they got it was just so awesome. Treating the massive amount of people, from the handicapped children in the two orphanages to infants and seniors was rewarding beyond words."

Dr. Craig Fishell gave a detailed account of his experience.

A few months back I became aware of a Chiromission trip to Dominican Republic. Several doctors would be going and adjusting thousands of people. On paper, it sounded good: an all-inclusive resort at a very good price, an excursion to a jungle, with the added bonus of high-volume chiropractic adjusting. I have been to many seminars, but nothing I have done can compare to this experience.

The agenda was clear. We would show up to this location at such and such time and adjust until there was no one left to adjust. Then we will eat lunch, go swimming, have dinner, wake up tomorrow, and do it again. The unknowns were, among others, how many people were going to come for adjustments, whether the river guides would be too weak or not speak English, whether we could break for lunch if we needed to keep going, and whether or not the driver going to be there. The mantra of Chiromission has become 'we will work it out when we get there,' and we did, because when something is pure, right, and completely driven by principle, nothing can block it. I went on this trip for one personal reason. I was looking for my heart.

The health paradigm in the United States is drug it, cut it, or tell them they are crazy, and the US is taking this paradigm to the entire world. Dominican Republic does not yet have a health paradigm. They do have a culture, and cultures supersede paradigms. As a result, most people in the DR were unaware of chiropractic. We told them that God created their bodies, with a nervous system that is protected by the spine. When we remove the interferences, the body heals, and most of these interferences are in the neck. This information was very well received in a culture that is 100 percent Catholic.

We were the first chiropractors that ever spoke to them. Being able to deliver an adjustment that was received as an instrument to connect them to their maker and bring them closer to their natural state, without by bias and untrue knowledge, was beautiful.

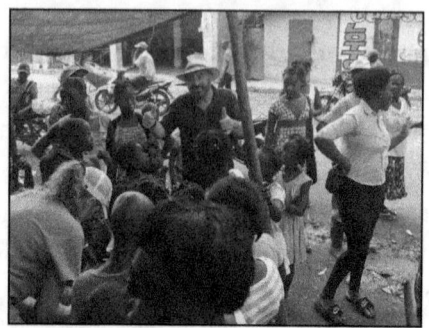

Adjusting a lot of children in Cap Haitien, Haiti.

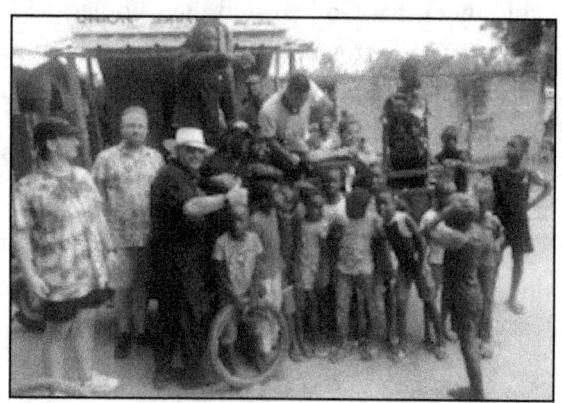

A union of saints helping people in Haiti.

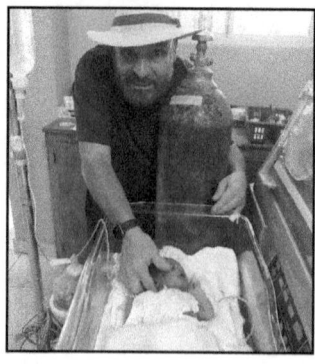

Adjusting a newborn at Univers Hospital.

PART II

The Mission Experience

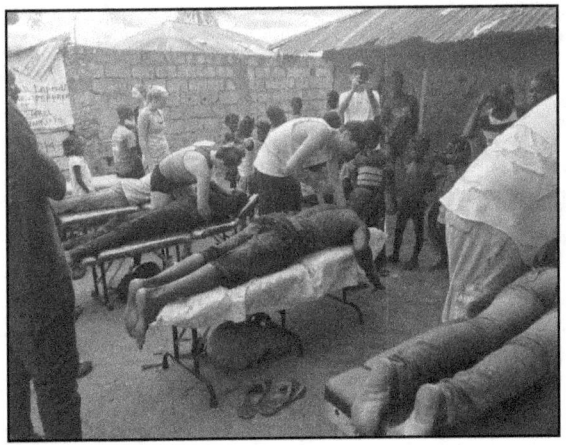

Terre Rouge, Haiti.

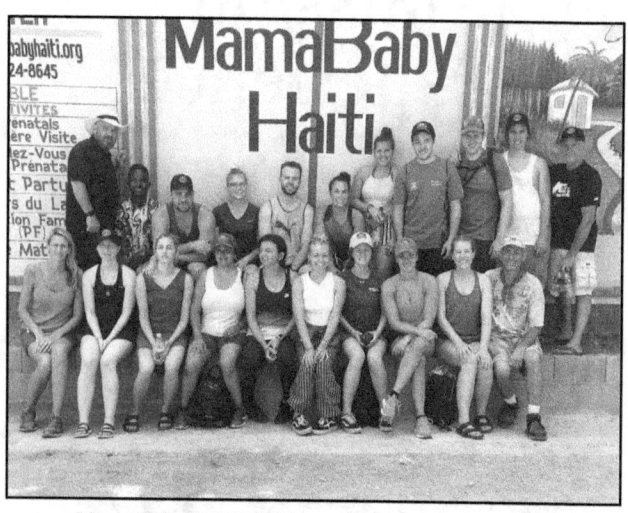

Mama Baby Haiti Birthing center Cap Hatian, Haiti.

CHAPTER 7

The Impact of Chiropractic Mission Trips

*Sometimes when we are generous in small,
barely detectable ways it can change
someone else's life forever.*

—MARGARET CHO

I have led nearly one hundred missions as of this writing in 2020, and every one of them has had major positive impacts on those we serve. I share the following stories with you to demonstrate how being a chiropractic missionary saves lives, relieves suffering, affects communities, and changes the lives of the missionaries themselves.

You may ask how a four-day experience can have such an impact on the patients and the chiropractic missionary. Why don't these kinds of things happen in everyday life? I believe it is because of three basic spiritual principles that occur with short-term missions experiences. The people of impoverished countries are waiting for a miracle to happen in their lives. When we arrive, they immediately comprehend that the intent of the chiropractor is to help them. Their spirit makes a connection with the spirit of the chiropractic missionary. The chiropractic missionary has an incredible spiritual connection with Universal Intelligence.

The role of the chiropractic adjustment is to restore the body's ability to heal itself. The chiropractic missionary attempts to restore the connection between the physical and the spiritual. The patient responds incredibly well because of the spiritual connection, the role of nature, and the removal of the vertebral subluxation. God rewards those who do His work. When we leave all of our conveniences and distractions behind to care for the poor and sick for a period of time, we are giving for the sake of giving, and we are God's servants.

God asks us to care for the less fortunate. When we answer this calling, we have an abundant life. Some people think this means material wealth, but it really means receiving the incredible joy and serenity we feel in meeting the needs of others who are desperate. Our service not only meets human needs, but it also reveals to God our true mission.

The spiritual individuality will present in a harmonious society of like-minded individuals. As a spiritual family, we share a conscious awareness between people. We recognize that each of our spirits is directly connected to God, and we can become consciously aware of that connection through D.D. Palmer's passages or through meditation. This approach encourages one to personally experience God instead of merely accepting the testimony of someone else.

After my first mission trip, I had a unique experience that I have never had before or since. I had visions that came to me during meditations of looking into the future. I would go into a deep hypnotic meditation and travel into the future, where I visualized all my goals becoming a reality. I had visions of many chiropractors and chiropractic students going on mission trips. In my visions, I raised objections as to why this could not be, yet for each objection, I received answers. For example, I thought, "The cost is too prohibitive." The answer I received was that money could be saved by renting houses and vans to transport people. Then I thought, "The people who most need to go on these trips are also least likely to spend a whole week." The answer to that was simple; they could get flights that left on Wednesday evening so they would miss only two days of work. Still another objection was, "People won't give up their conveniences." The answer to this was short and to the point: "You did." Last, I wondered, "How will they know what an impact Chiromissions can have?" The answer was, "You will tell them." I now believe that many of those chiropractors whom I saw in those visions represent the future chiropractic leaders.

My hope in sharing the following stories is that they will inspire you to create your own missions.

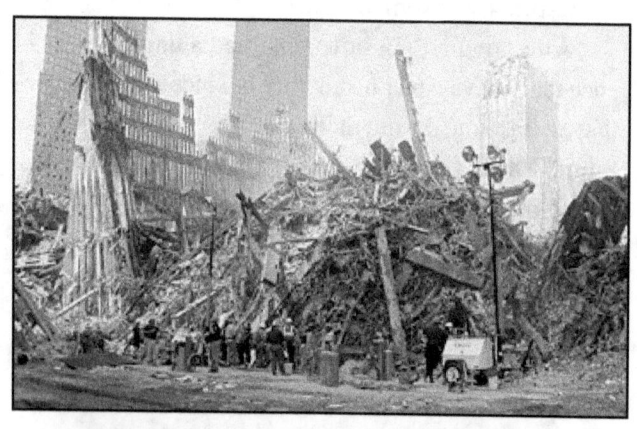

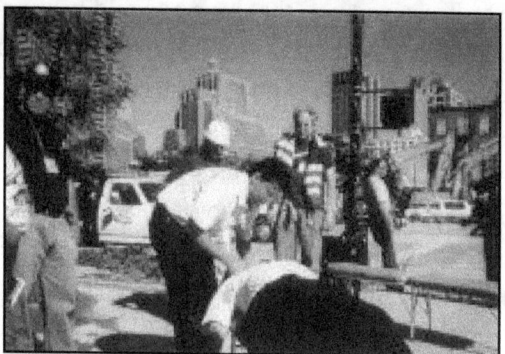

2001 Dr. Glenn Scarpelli adjusting at Ground Zero.
Dr. Scarpelli was Vice President while I was
President of the NY Chiropractic Council.

CHAPTER 8

My First Chiropractic Mission Trip, 9/11

Charity sees the need, not the cause.

—GERMAN PROVERB

New York City is the place where I was born, grew up, and opened my chiropractic practice. In 2001 I was on the executive board of the New York Chiropractic Council and later became its president. On October 25, 2001, the New York Chiropractic Council bestowed on me the coveted Chiropractor of the Year Beacon Award, given for outstanding and unselfish service to chiropractic.

It should have been a great year for me, but many of our patients and friends were dead. It was the worst year ever for our families and friends. On September 11, 2001, our city was attacked, and I entered into my first mission trip.

The telephone rang. It was Dr. Ellen Coyne, president of the New York Chiropractic Council. Our city had been struck with the world's worst act of terrorism ever. "Oh my God, we need to work with Mayor Giuliani," she said. "We need to work with Senator Clinton, Governor Pataki, and the President." I agreed. "We need to bring chiropractors down to the site to help in whatever way we can." "I agree!" I replied. In that moment, Dr. Coyne created the chiropractic relief effort at Ground Zero, and I was her trusted friend and executive officer.

She was amazing and extremely organized. We composed several letters that we dispatched to Mayor Giuliani, Governor Pataki, Senator Hillary Clinton, President George Bush, the New York State Board of Chiropractic, and many others.

The next day, Dr. Gary DiBenedetto was serving at the Ground Zero site. Suddenly, the police arrived and began to escort Dr. DiBenedetto from the area. Two fireman who Dr. Gary had previously adjusted stepped in and told the cops, "We need the chiropractors here!" Dr. Gary relayed the message to Dr. Coyne, and then we spent many hours on the phone.

Within a few hours, Dr. Coyne had scheduled a meeting with the American Red Cross officials. The Red Cross then sanctioned chiropractic as a vital part of the recovery efforts. Thanks to the efforts of Dr. Gary DiBenedetto, Dr. Ellen Coyne, and many others at the New York Chiropractic Council, we created a bond with the Red Cross to staff the Ground Zero respite centers with chiropractors. For the first time in chiropractic history, we officially collaborated with this great humanitarian organization.

Many of my friends were first responders. In the succeeding days, chiropractors from state, national, and international chiropractic associations participated. My job was to work with the Red Cross to photograph and credential every chiropractic volunteer serving at Ground Zero.

Many of the volunteers, rescue workers, and others had their first experience with chiropractic and chiropractors. They met with the most dedicated chiropractors from the profession that could be put together in one place. To this day, many of these people and their families continue under chiropractic care.

During the nine months that our doctors were there, they donated more than $1.5 million in chiropractic services. One thousand five hundred chiropractors provided incredible care to approximately 500 police officers, fire fighters, and other volunteers at the five respite centers.

Chiropractors came from all over the country, including Hawaii and Alaska. They all came to serve chiropractic at the Ground Zero Relief sites. I frequently visited the respite centers in an administrative capacity. I remember attending a mass one evening at the Iron Cross. The Iron Cross was made from iron beams that came from the twin towers' north building. As I sat and prayed, I thought about how spiritual the place was. I later found out that it was a sacred place for all the Ground Zero relief team.

One day, after leaving the many volunteers who were serving at the respite centers, I went to the Iron Cross to take a break from the exhausting work of caring for hundreds of traumatized people. From my position I could see across the entire site, all the way to St. Paul's Chapel. The terrain looked so strange and unusual, like a setting from another planet. I felt as if I were on the moon, with a never-ending task in front of me.

Of all the respite centers, St. Paul's was my favorite. After the attacks of September 11, 2001, St. Paul's Chapel, which sits directly across the street from the World Trade Center site, suffered no physical damage. On September 12, Lyndon Harris, the clergy on staff at Trinity and St. Paul's, arrived at St. Paul's Chapel. He was sure that there would be large-scale destruction. He was shocked to find that inside the building, the church was in perfect order, but the exterior surface of the sanctuary and the churchyard were covered in ash. Engineers inspected the building and pronounced it sound. The Ground Zero respite center was opened.

Many first responders, firefighters, military, construction workers, clergy, and other professionals came to St. Paul's for meals, beds, rest, and chiropractic adjustments. I recall one evening when I was bringing a new volunteer doctor to St. Paul's. A police officer approached and asked if I could provide him with an adjustment. I had already adjusted many of his friends. After I cared for the officer, many other police officers arrived. One by one they put their guns under our adjusting tables and got adjusted. We adjusted them all in two hours. Only then did I get a chance to show the new doc around. Moments later, I stopped and reflected. I was so honored to be able to help my city. I broke down and started to cry.

This was my first mission trip, and it had set the tone for all of the mission trips I subsequently created and administered.

What follows are the stories of many of my good friends and classmates who served in the relief effort at Ground Zero, many of whom were first responders. The events of that day were some of the most traumatic that our country has ever suffered. The doctors served with a desire to help their fellow countrymen and to serve their country. Their stories are now part of American history.

RICHARD GORGO JR., DC

When he heard the news of the disaster, my friend and colleague Richard Gorgo Jr., DC, knew he had to do something. He lived three hours from New York City, but he packed up some medical supplies, his chiropractic table, and all the bedding and pillows he could find and headed toward the city. Amazingly, he was allowed to pass into the no-go zone when he told an officer that he was a doctor and was there to help.

He headed toward the Jacob Javits Center, which was one of five respite areas that were rapidly being set up across the area. The Javits Center was "full of search-and-rescue teams that were still pouring in from all around the country and even from around the world," he said. "Then the patients started coming."

After working almost day and night for the first couple of days, Dr. Gorgo was given permission to head through five checkpoints to "the Pile," the smoking and twisted remains of what had been a tower of the World Trade Center just days before. The devastation was everywhere, and so were exhausted and stressed workers and volunteers. Dr. Gorgo said, "Just before I left [to go to the Pile], I remember seeing a US marshal passed out on some folding chairs. She had been up for over forty hours. I remember handing her a pillow."

After working his way through the bureaucracy that surrounds disasters no matter the magnitude, Dr. Gorgo finally made it to the Pile, heart of the tragedy that was to be forever known as 9/11. He recalled, "Our first impression was the smell; oh, how I will never forget that smell. Beyond that, our inability to see due to the thick smoke and all the different uniforms rushing around created a sensation that was unreal. We always said it felt like we were on a movie set where King Kong was battling Godzilla in Manhattan."

He entered St. Peter's Church, which had also been set up as a respite center. As he set up his table between the pews, he noticed the thick layer of dust that covered everything. He said, "I remember walking in that dust; it looked like we were on the surface of the moon. I was later told that the church had been completely locked and sealed during the towers' collapse, yet great amounts of dust still made it in."

He went on to describe the mood that enveloped the entire city. "The attitude at the site can't be emphasized enough. It was solemn yet busy, but with an air of hope. There was no smiling, no emotion; just work—and you dared not have a camera. I saw a news cameraman trying to sneak around, and they picked him up and threw him out of the site. This was not a place of discovery, journalism, or interest—not then. This was the place where so many of these people had lost someone. These men lost brothers and sisters. They were working nonstop for days."

Dr. Gorgo befriended Officer Gail Imhauser, a transit cop who, like all of the professionals and volunteers at work at the Pile, had been pressed into a job that no one would have chosen. She started calling Dr. Gorgo to visit fellow police officers who couldn't take leave from their work "or even remove their bulletproof vests." He met those heroes in "building lobbies, alleyways, and even dining halls" to provide them on-the-spot treatment.

Dr. Gorgo relayed a particularly poignant story of "a passed-out fireman lying on an I-beam. Smoke was pouring out all around him. I shook him and told him

I was a doctor. I asked him to come back with me to the makeshift clinic we had made in the church. He didn't want anything to do with me; he did not want to be taken off the Pile and away from his brothers, whose rescue alarms we could hear going off underneath the wreckage. I expressed to him that I was a chiropractor and that I might be able to help him. I brought him back to the church, assessed and adjusted him. He got a burst of energy and thanked me."

Shortly after his arrival, Dr. Gorgo had treated over 100 people. He later noted, "The police, firefighters, US marshals, military police, FEMA teams, city cleanup crews, transit authority workers, engineers, city council members, and on and on chose chiropractic care."

Dr. Gorgo ultimately spent three months working onsite after the towers fell.(You can read more of Dr. Gorgo's story in his article "Where Were You When the World Stopped Turning?" in *Dynamic Chiropractic*, September 9, 2011, vol. 29, no. 19.)

JOHN PRZYBYLAK, DC

My friend, colleague, and fellow chiropractor Dr. John Przybylak and his wife, Dr. Jessica D'Amore, went to Ground Zero on September 31, 2001, twenty days after the worst terrorist attack in America's history. As they drove through the city and through the same security scrutiny as their colleague Dr. Gorgo had, they were finally directed to the Pile. Once they arrived at the Murray Street Respite Center at St. John's University, they immediately got to work, treating people for the next six hours straight.

Dr. John observed, "The firefighters were deeply stricken. They had lost so many in the tragedy; 343 members of NYFD [had] perished. The blunted stare of a man in shock three weeks after the loss is an ominous site. No emotion showed through the pall-like masks each wore."

He went on to describe the surreal feeling that cast an indelible pall over the Pile. "A particular sound . . . stood significantly higher above the din—it was a siren. That shrieking whistle would decrescendo, and the silence would become deafening while the siren took a breath. . . . It was not a call to flee. Instead, we all gathered in line at the street's side to observe a motorcade of police cycles followed by two police cars and an ambulance. The flashing lights and siren horn were acknowledged by a devoted army of workers who solemnly stood at attention and saluted the ambulance rolling by. Another victim found in the wreckage. One could not hold the gripping emotion as a fellow citizen is transported to the morgue. We joined in this ceremony, and also saluted where we stood."

Dr. John later explained that the chiropractic care that takes place after a disaster is different from that in an office. The stresses are unique, the nature of the workers' backbreaking work was extreme, and the emotional toll on the volunteers and professionals alike rapidly mounted. An undefined fear lay over everyone "like an unwanted guest."

Dr. John told of another chiropractor, Dr. Donna Mutter, who said, "These brave men and women were so armored, wrapped in large overalls and boots, and equipped with ropes, lights, guns, knives, cables, hard hats, gloves, and masks. They were covered in dirt and cuts and dust. Their bodies were exhausted from lack of sleep; emotions were raw from so much loss . . . loss of friends, brothers, and sisters, and from the frustration that no one was coming out alive. Recovering body parts of the dead and a few whole bodies was a living hell. The dust on their cloths and boots contained the ashes of the countless dead. I looked at my hands and realized these hands were touching ashes of the dead."

Dr. John noted that the most common reaction from people who were getting adjustments was simply being able to breathe freely. He watched as his wife, Dr. Jessi, adjusted a firefighter, and then witnessed the man undergo a dramatic change as the adjustment brought him "out of his personal hell." The firefighter said, "This is the first deep breath I've taken in a long time." The second most notable reaction was relaxation. The doctors could tell when this happened "by a good healthy sigh. They wanted to sleep." The third and perhaps most notable reaction was when someone would get off the table and begin telling a story about what had happened to them or a loved one. They needed to talk, and they needed a hug. They got both.

Dr. John stayed at Ground Zero for two months, selflessly dedicating himself to the relief efforts that were so important to the well-being of the boots-on-the-ground workers. (You can read more of Dr. John's story, "Chiropractic Rescue and the American Tragedy: The Chiropractic Relief Effort at Ground Zero," at http://www.chiropraxiswedel.de/files/Chiropractic_Rescue_and_the_American_Tragedy.pdf.)

DR. GARY DEUTCHMAN AND DR. HOLLY TIDWELL

My friend and colleague Dr. Gary Deutchman also felt called to help at Ground Zero within days of the disaster. He went ready to lend a hand in whatever way he could. None of us could foresee how important chiropractic was to become in the days, weeks, and months after 9/11 as members of our profession continued to coalesce around the much-needed respite centers.

The first chiropractors who poured into devastated parts of the city didn't have official permission to be there as service providers, but that didn't stop these incredible souls from talking their way into the heart of the activity. Dr. Deutchman was one of those need-driven volunteers, ready to set to work in the midst of the unimaginable. He recalled, "As the crowds of policemen, soldiers, firemen, and tradesmen came out of the destruction zone after hours of digging, passing buckets, and other more technical jobs, I would shout out, 'Chiropractic over here, who's next for chiropractic?' Some people looked at me like I had two heads. Others would come over, so thankful we were there." He treated several hundred people over the next fifteen hours.

Dr. Deutchman eventually made his way to the Red Cross ship that was docked at Battery Park. He continued to focus on providing treatment to as many people as he could. He said, "I brought my portable table over to the ship and set up in the middle of the busiest area. I went up to one really large fireman and asked him if he wanted to get adjusted. I told him once everyone saw him get adjusted there would be a line, so he should be the first to get adjusted. He agreed, and the whole main deck was watching this guy in a white lab coat (me) adjust this big fireman.... I made my adjustment, and the guy got up and said, 'Wow. That was amazing.' For the next few hours, I had a line of people from every type of law enforcement agency and fire department from here to Canada waiting in line. Many of the people had never had a chiropractic adjustment [before]."

Dr. Holly Tidwell, who also was hard at work near Ground Zero, acknowledged the physical and emotional toll the work was taking on the chiropractors. She said, "It is admittedly sometimes hard to go back, but then you realize what they are going through, and you want to." She also pointed out that the canine searchers were working just as hard as anyone else. She said, "The dogs come back exhausted as well, and we have DC's to adjust them, and then they get massaged, too." (To read more on the stories of Dr. Deutchman, Dr. Tidwell, and others who volunteered at Ground Zero after 9/11, please see "Chiropractors Lend a Hand at Ground

Zero," https://www.anchorchiropractic.net/2019/09/10/chiropractors-lend-a-hand-at-ground-zero/.)

The brave and selfless chiropractors who came to the 9/11 tragedy to provide support for the hundreds of search-and-rescue workers who were working around the clock became a vital part of the operation. Our work later was recognized by organizations and people all over the country. Our relief effort also became a model for how chiropractors can provide a significant asset in times of disaster and trauma. We will not forget.

While our work at Ground Zero and the Pile wasn't officially a mission trip, I have always considered it so, as so many of us were spiritually called to volunteer our services during one of the greatest tragedies our country has ever suffered. As I look back, I remember the wonderful people who I met. There were phenomenal doctors, nurses, Red Cross volunteers, and chiropractors who worked to help people twenty-four hours a day for nine months. During this time, I witnessed unimaginable things.

I also saw healthcare professionals with loving hearts who were the most competent people you could ever meet. I met many people in the mental health field. These skilled professionals helped many people deal with their 9/11 post-trauma.

Perhaps one of the greatest lessons that has come from 9/11 is the tremendous debt of gratitude that we owe our nation's firefighters, police, and paramedics, men and women who are all too easily taken for granted, yet they continue to serve and protect us every day. What is perhaps even more remarkable was how we as a nation rallied together and supported their efforts.

Virtually everyone, young and old, pitched in to some degree, offering what they could: their time, their talent, their energy, and their prayers. This unified effort brought our nation to a new level.

There is no question that the magnitude of the tragedy that occurred on September 11, 2001, was exactly what the terrorists were looking for, but what they probably didn't forecast was the altruistic backlash that rose up because of it. No, they didn't tear us down —they built us up. They made us stronger than we had ever been as a nation. They rekindled the spirit of patriotism that our founding fathers must have had. The words "United States," "In God We Trust," and "God Bless America" now have a deeper, more emotional tie than they ever had before for most of us.

I am proud to say that the 1,776-foot-tall Freedom Tower and the National September 11 Memorial & Museum now stand in the place of the twin towers. I recommend visiting the 9/11 museum, which honors the many victims of the attacks and all those who risked their lives to rescue and save others.

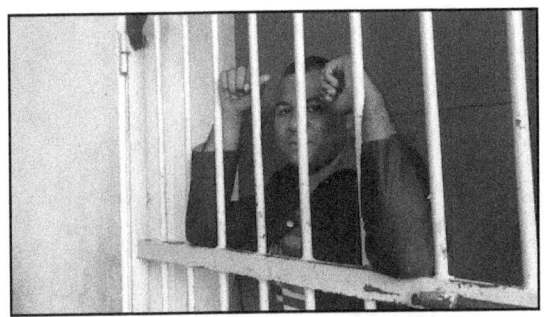

Adjusting prisoners in one of the largest prisons in the Dominican Republic.

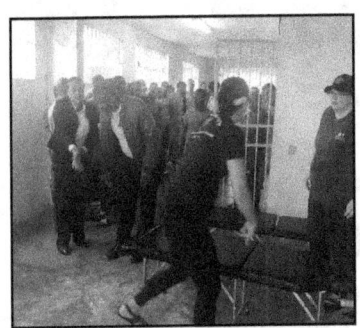

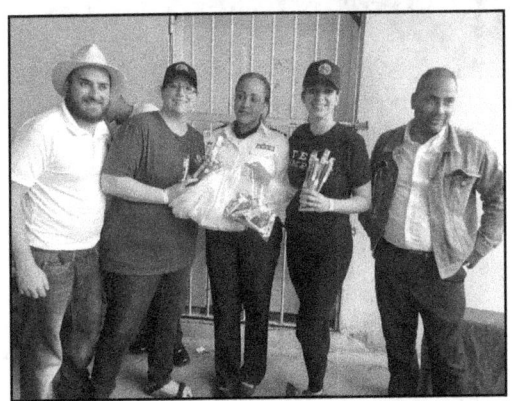

Bobbi Joy Voermans, DC; Lauryn Brunclik, DC and Carlos Casanova, DC adjusting in one of the largest prisons in the Dominican Republic. I did a facebook live as we adjusted the prisoners.

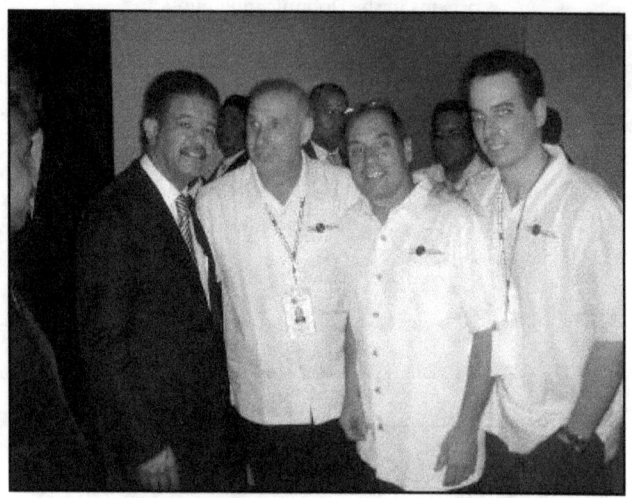

Todd Herold, DC; JC Doornick and I with the President of the Dominican Republic Leonel Fernandez in 2008

CHAPTER 9

Mission Trip to Dominican Republic, March 2007

We are made wise not by the recollection of our past, but by the responsibility for our future.

—GEORGE BERNARD SHAW

In March 2007, a team chiropractor missionaries went on a Chiromission to Dominican Republic through the Mission Life International. Our mission was to serve the people of Dominican Republic with love and compassion, to promote chiropractic, and to adjust all those who are subluxated throughout the country, where resources are so terribly limited. Our intention was to create a free chiropractic clinic for the poor.

We arrived with eighteen chiropractors and twenty chiropractic students from Life Chiropractic College. On our first day there, we wanted to liberate our fears before starting to adjust, so we created a fear challenge.

It began with a hike across a wide and rough river. We walked five at a time, connected to one another by our folded arms. If one of us broke loose, the whole group could be trouble. Luckily, we had guides behind us to save any of the fallen.

As we crossed the river, we encountered a strong current that made us drift downstream, but we finally arrived to the other side. Was that a snake? Or could it be a wild boar? No, it was just one of the guides playing a joke on us. Our group of forty proceeded through the jungle, hugging the side of a stronger, narrower river. We crossed over that river nine or ten times during the next hour.

We arrived at a huge waterfall. Were we crazy? As we attempted to climb the falls, many of us fell back five or six feet into the whirlpool of water. The guides placed our feet on treacherous and slippery rocks as they pushed, pulled, and lifted us up the falls. The water rushed over us with a current so strong it could rip a 250-pound man away from the guides.

Our guides were short, small, and light, but they could lift men twice their size as if they were feathers. They could swim like sharks and climb like monkeys. This was fortunate for two of the women with us. Doreen slipped off the falls, and one of the guides dove off a cliff and pulled her out of the thunderous and extreme rapids.

As we approached the fourth level of the waterfall (there are twenty-seven), Morgan was bumped by a guide and fell into the rapids. She grabbed onto a guide, and they both went flying down the rapids. Fortunately, JC was able to stop them and pull them out. At that point, the guides forbade us to move on. It had been raining for two weeks, and the water was at its highest level. The last time we had a team here and did the challenge, we made it to the twentieth level, and it was easier than the first three levels on this day.

We had to turn back, and the only way down was to jump from cliffs into small pools of water. The first cliff was an easy ten feet. The next cliff was a little more challenging at twelve feet. It took some people more than twenty minutes to jump. To get down to the first level, we could jump a ten-foot cliff, or we could face all fears and jump off a sixty-six-foot cliff. Since this was my third fear challenge and I enjoy high jumping, I had been wanting to take the big jump. In the past, the guides would never let me. On this trip, I made them an offer they could not refuse. I would double their tip.

Since I have experience jumping and diving off cliffs, I knew that you just have to do it. The longer you stand on the cliff, the harder it becomes. So when the guides gave me the go-ahead, I went for it. It was a long drop, and I had to land in a very small area. What a rush! After I made it, I looked back up, and boy, was I surprised. I saw fifteen chiropractic missionaries lined up for the big plunge. It took some of them a long time to purge their fears, but they all did.

The next day we headed to our mission at the Casa de Oracion, the Healing House. When our thirty-eight chiropractors and students arrived, Sor (Sister) Teodora and many other nuns met us. Sor Teodora must be Mother Teresa's sister. The love that emanates from her is beyond description. When we presented her with 150 million pesos in donations, tears flowed as strong as the river on the previous today.

Amore, love, and compassion were requirements for this beautiful mission, and we received so much back. Our hands-on miracle healers were sent to sixteen remote locations, including orphanages. We adjusted nine thousand people in three days. One group, a chiropractor and two chiropractic students, were sent to a location that also had a medical mission going on at the same time. The medical mission was giving out drugs like candy. The chiropractic missionaries told the people, "The power that made the body heals the body." Hundreds of people switched lines for adjustments. A riot broke out, the National Guard was called in, and the chiropractic missionaries were put out to the street. On the street, they adjusted hundreds of people.

On the last day of the mission trip, we were enlightened once again. We sat around a bonfire on the beach, and each chiropractic missionary told of their experience. We all had one thing in common: we were there to serve with adjustments, hugs, love, and compassion to help alleviate the suffering of the poorest of the poor.

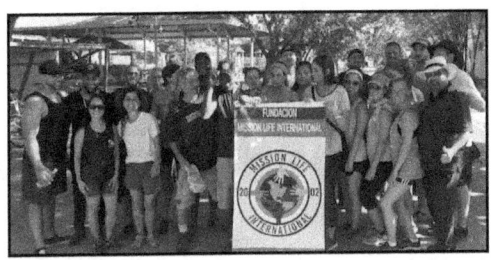

Wonderful mission work in the D.R. 2019. Daniel Pichette, DC with Henri Rosenblum led a number of Life University Students in Dajabon, Dominican Republic.

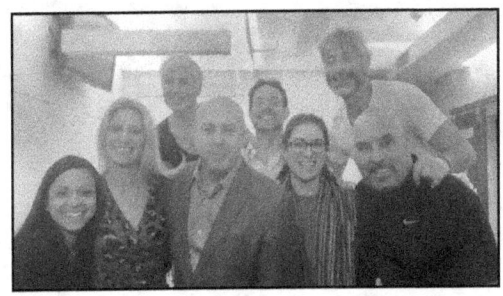

Stu Warner, DC and Theresa Warner, DC at our District 4 NY Chiropractic meeting.

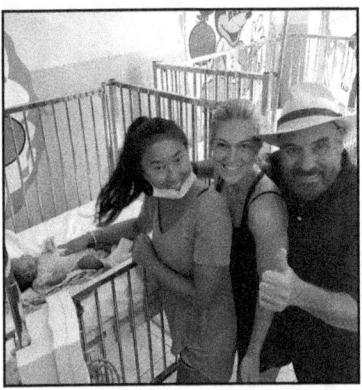

With Clara White, DC and Veronica Gobeil, DC. Adjusting newborns at Univers Hospital. Ouanaminthe, Haiti. 2017

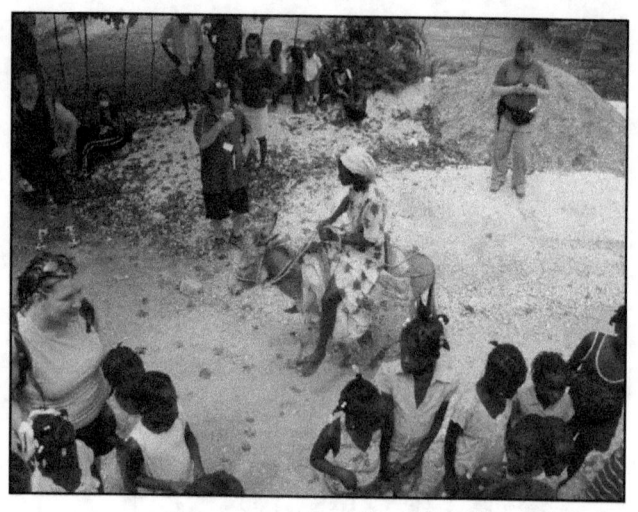

A few days after the earthquake in Haiti January 2010.

CHAPTER 10

Mission Trip to Haiti, April 2008

Seek out that particular mental attribute which makes you feel most deeply and vitally alive, along with which comes the inner voice which says, "This is the real me," and when you have found that attitude, follow it.

—WILLIAM JAMES

A month after our March 2008 mission trip, a new team of chiropractors and students headed back Dominican Republic, and this time our Chiromissions team was also going to Haiti. There had never been a chiropractor in Ouanaminthe, Haiti.

Our purpose on this trip was to educate hospitals, schools, and pastors about chiropractic. Since Todd and I had gotten there early, we also had to prepare for the mission and for the arrival of the sixty-five chiropractors and students.

On Sunday, March 30, 2008, we received the call out of nowhere. The President of Dominican Republic, Leonel Fernandez, was to be at a press conference at six o'clock that evening to inaugurate a brand new hospital that we were working with to implement chiropractic and proactive and preventative health care. Todd's brother in-law worked security for the President and had facilitated the meeting.

We waited four hours because the President was mobbed with press, and his motorcade was slowed down by traffic. Todd's brother-in-law then came, grabbed us by the arm, and insisted we follow him. Some doors opened, and we walked into an enormous press conference with thousands of people in attendance. As we marched into the large arena with music blaring, people were chanting, "Presidente Leonel, Presidente Leonel." People were reaching, grabbing, and trying to touch us as we proceeded up to the dais. The temperature felt like 110 degrees as the press were taking pictures. This was a nationally televised event, and we realized that we were walking into it with the President and his cabinet.

We stood in the front with the Secret Service agents in a private viewing area for another two hours. Todd and I gave them all adjustments while JC photographed. After the President was whisked away, we were maneuvered through side doors by security and found ourselves in a private area, where our meeting finally happened.

It was midnight as the President mentioned in perfect English how excited and thankful he was of our work here. I said that we wanted to build a chiropractic school here in Dominican Republic, and he said, "Go for it."

The next day, Todd and I, along with mission leaders JC and Jason O'Connor, spoke to group of over fifty medical residents, recent medical graduates, and the heads of several medical departments at Morillo King Hospital in La Vega, Dominican Republic. The lecture was an introduction to chiropractic. We explained the chiropractor's role as primary health care providers centered on vertebral subluxation detection and correction. We also discussed the possibility of bringing chiropractic to the country on a permanent basis.

On this Chiromissions trip, Mission Life International led a team of thirty-two chiropractors and thirty-one chiropractic students to the jungles and remote villages of this island of two nations. We had more than thirty teams, each one consisting of a chiropractor, a chiropractic student, and a mission guide. We were accompanied by a film team and were verified for a world record with Record Holders Republic.[3]

On this mission trip, we brought the healing power of chiropractic to hundreds upon hundreds of Haitians in the town of Ouanaminthe and thousands upon thousands of people in multiple Dominican Republic

---

[3] Record Holders Republic, http://www.recordholdersrepublic.co.uk/world-record-holders/545/peter-morgan.aspx

cities, villages, and hilltop towns. Todd and JC led fifteen teams in four regions, and I led ten teams in another four. The rippling effects of this chiropractic pebble dropping into the pond were just beginning.

Todd and I had recently been in Dominican Republic to meet President Leonel Fernandez's cabinet and other political leaders to talk about chiropractic's role in helping the people recover from the devastation by Hurricane Olga hurricane three months before. We also met the Speaker of the House of Representatives, the Honorable Julio Cesar Valentine, Senator Dominguez-Vrito, and other political leaders. The meeting was organized by Mr. Benedicto Bernandez, the coordinator of the 168 members of the House of Representatives.

We were also welcomed at the New York Dominican Republic Consulate by the chief council and staff. It was the first-ever chiropractic symposium in the inner sanctum of the Grand Counsel's office, and included politicians dignitaries, and media. More than ten pastors from Dominican Republic were also present at the historic televised event. Special thanks to Gregorio Malena, Vice Consul for orchestrating this event.

Todd and I then went on a tour of the area, which had been destroyed as a result of the recent hurricanes. We saw the result of Mother Nature's terrible wrath. We were in the home of a ninety-seven-year-old woman named Carmen. When the storms hit overnight, she found herself neck high in six feet of muddy water in her bedroom. To save her, her family brought a horse into her casita—a home the size of a small US living room—and dragged her out. Later, when Todd and I asked her what she thought of the experience, she had no complaints and thanked God for all that she still had.

Our team spent time meeting with the directors of the mainstream hospitals to discuss the possibility of bringing chiropractic to the country on a permanent basis. Dominican Republic government and medical profession have embraced the concept 100 percent. We were asked to deliver a presentation on subluxation based chiropractic philosophy and to administer chiropractic care to all of the patients of a major Dominican Republic hospital.

We wanted to begin a proactive healthcare strategy so that we could begin to apply our philosophy, as we saw the value in teaching our patients to maximize their health potential and avoid disease in the first place. We took the necessary steps to get the wheels rolling for the first-ever chiropractic school in the DR.

It's Up to You

One song can spark a moment,
One flower can wake the dream.
One tree can start a forest,
One bird can herald spring.
One smile begins a friendship,
One handclasp lifts a soul.
One star can guide a ship at sea,
One word can frame the goal.
One vote can change a nation,
One sunbeam lights a room.
One candle wipes out darkness,
One laugh will conquer gloom.
One step must start each journey,
One word must start each prayer.
One hope will raise our spirits,
One touch can show you care.
One voice can speak with wisdom,
One heart can know what's true,
One life can make a difference,
You see, it's up to you.

—AUTHOR UNKNOWN

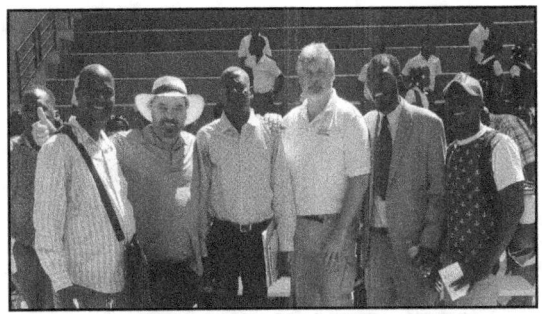

Alex Thoni, Samuel Garcon, Rob Scott, DC and I in a meeting with the President and VP of the Cap Hatian music school.

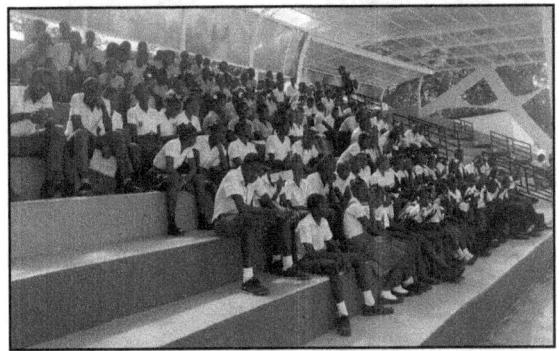

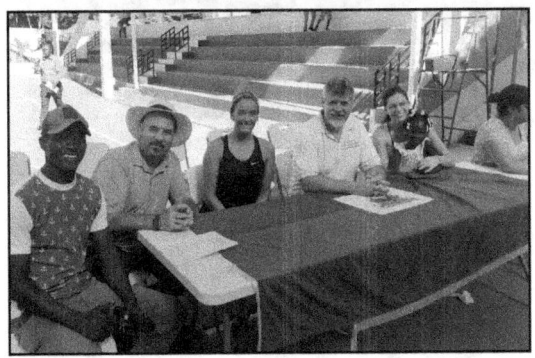

Rob Scott, DC President of Life University addressed the top high school students of Haiti in Ouanaminthe, Haiti

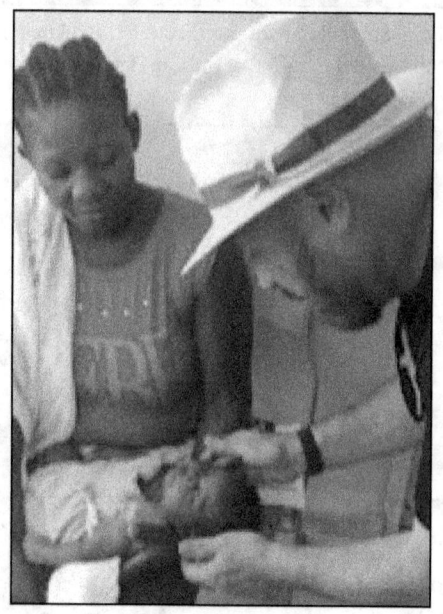

A beautiful baby. 2016

CHAPTER 11

Mission Trip to Haiti, June 2008

Whoever renders service to many puts himself in line for greatness—great wealth, great return, great satisfaction, great reputation, and great joy

—JIM ROHN

Since I had been to Haiti with a church mission group, I organized the Chiromissions Haiti expedition and led this brave team of chiropractors. Other mission leaders were David Hecht, DC, from New York, and John Palmer, student leader and chiropractic student at Life University.

There was a lot of uncertainty from both Haiti and Chiromissions as to how this mission trip was going to work. I was organizing with people who had never received an adjustment and did not know what chiropractic was. I also don't speak Creole, so there was a language gap. I was nervous and apprehensive regarding our physical safety. I was concerned about the sanitary conditions. However, since our mission was so important, I was willing to try. I trusted that God would see that things worked out.

The expansion to Haiti fit nicely into Chiromission's desire to bring the benefits of chiropractic to people who cannot afford healthcare. During our chiropractic mission trip in October 2007, I was introduced by a Dominican friend to Rezene Tesfamariam, director of Plan Haiti International. Plan Haiti has donated $350,000 toward the construction of a kindergarten at Institution Univers, a school of fifteen hundred students in Ouanaminthe. Understanding the objectives of Chiromissions, Rezene introduced me to Hugues Bastien, the founder of Institution Univers.

Things usually look ugly before they get better. Our team almost decided to turn back when we got to the border and were told we couldn't take our rental car across. We were weary, hungry, and sweaty from our long trip from Puerto Plata to the Haitian border, not to mention nervous, anxious, and apprehensive. We received lots of offers from strange people to watch our rental car while we went across the river to Haiti. Images of returning to a dismantled vehicle, or no vehicle at all, ran through our minds. We couldn't reach our contact person, Hugues Bastien, on the phone, and we were stranded for hours.

Little children were coming from Haiti begging for money. Several of them approached our car windows, and we could see their skin riddled with all sorts of skin diseases, teeth that were decayed to the roots, and the filthy rags they wearing for clothes. We could see across the border to the outskirts of a very poor town with very sparse vegetation, and garbage everywhere.

Our team began looking for every reason not to go forward, but just as we were beginning to make plans to leave, we received a call from Mr. Bastien. He confirmed the fact that we couldn't bring the vehicle across the border. We didn't feel any more secure when he told us that he might have a place where it could be left. When Dave asked if it would be safe, Mr. Bastien just replied, "Trust me," followed by an unsettling laugh. We really had no other choice, so we left our car and keys, and our team hopped into Mr. Bastien's four-wheel drive van and crossed into Ouanaminthe.

Our team of chiropractic missionaries were so happy that we endured the hardships and carried on with the mission. We would have missed out on a great opportunity to serve, and the people who were expecting us would have been severely disappointed.

We finally arrived at the medical center where we were going to give adjustments. The staff had scheduled appointments for us, just like a regular office. We were four chiropractors, and they had scheduled a hundred patients per hour.

People showed up consistently throughout the day. We worked nonstop, overseeing all the scheduled patients plus walk-ins for those days that we were in

Ouanaminthe. Each member of our team worked a solid twelve hours or more. To help with the language barrier, we had translators who educated all the people about the chiropractic story as they waited. They placed emphasis on the vitalistic principle that "the power that made the body heals the body."

The facility at Universe Medical Centre was built for all types of health providers who donate their time and talents to help the people. Our team learned that the there was only one health provider in the region, a medical doctor. He was able to spend only 25 percent of his time spent seeing patients because of the administrative responsibilities he also carried.

Our guide and contact person, Hugues Bastien, was one of twelve children. A well-educated gentleman, he receiving an advanced engineering degree in college. His entire family immigrated to the United States, but Hugues had a dream to build an educational center in his hometown. The educators at the center would teach children how to prepare for, create, and take advantage of opportunities when they come along. Little by little, Hugues built the school. In the beginning, he saved money by working as a taxi driver in New York. Slowly but surely he worked and toiled on his dream. Finally, Hugues's dream came to fruition, and now there is a stunning educational facility with one thousand six hundred students. Another facility was also nearing completion; it would be able to house teams of fifty to sixty doctors who could stay for a week or longer.

Hugues's engineering background allowed him to turn his vision into reality, and Chiromissions was able to share in his joy as the fruits of his labor were beginning to show. We were tremendously blessed by what we received from the experience in Ouanaminthe. We went with one purpose: to give of ourselves. We will never forget this!

In Dominican Republic, thirty teams were stationed all over the country. Many of the chiropractors were on their first mission trip, but they all prepared for an incredibly powerful week of love and service, giving God's greatest gift to man: chiropractic. Teams were located in mountain villages, in city ghettos, in orphanages, nursing homes, prisons, baseball fields, and villages that had been devastated by a recent hurricane. Some teams adjusted as many as a thousand people in a day. The average team adjusted four hundred people a day. Almost every team adjusted every student in every local school.

All types of people presented to our teams. There were newborn infants clutching their mothers' breasts, people over a hundred years old, people with hatchet wounds, people on crutches and in wheelchairs, a woman with bleeding goiters, people with huge tumors, priests, pastors, ministers, curios passersby who wandered over—an endless procession of people with all kinds of ailments. They were all looking for a miracle from the chiropractic miracle workers. The chiropractors analyzed and adjusted solely for the purpose of removing nerve interference. As D.D. Palmer wrote, "Our mission is to reunite the physical with the spiritual."

I had been stationed at this exact site on the last mission trip and saw the pastor whom I had eaten dinner with at his house, where I spent a night. We spoke about our wonderful night, and I thanked him for helping us with our mission trip. As I was leaving, three women asked if I could adjust them. I told them that this was not my station and the chiropractors who were working there would take care of them. One of them replied, "Oh, no, Doctor, you have to take care of me. The last time you were here, you created a miracle in my life."

The other two women had the same story. One of the women had had a tumor that went away, another had a goiter that went away, and the third had digestive problems that were completely gone. I said that I did not perform any miracles, that I am an instrument of the universe here to remove vertebral subluxations, which allows the body to work better. But, of course, I had to adjust these three women. Each adjustment was accompanied by a hug, and the love just poured forth.

I stayed a while longer and helped the two other chiropractors, because hundreds of people had come two hours early and were waiting. People cried, laughed, smiled, and grinned after they got adjusted, but they all respected the sacred art of adjusting the spine.

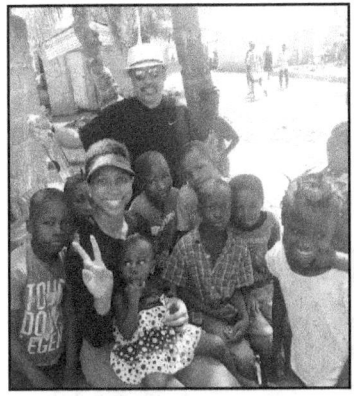

Shekinah Sharpe fell in love with our kids at the orphanage.

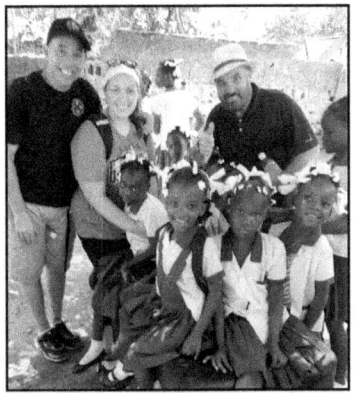

Stephen Simonetti, DC and I are adjusting a lot of children. Shayna Gorman is a great chiropractic assistant.

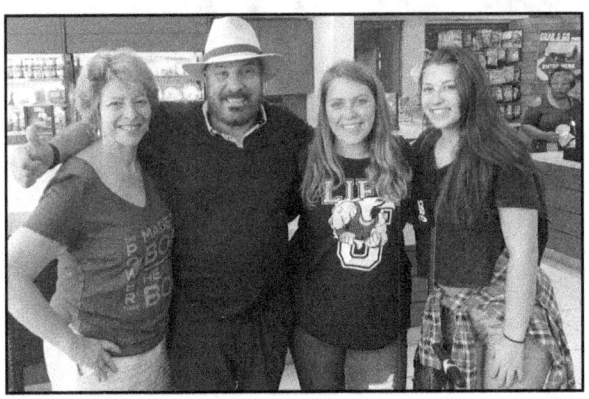

Sharon Gorman, DC; Sophie Gorman and Shayna Gorman met me at the Miami airport before our 90 minute flight to Cap Hatian. Sharon quickly became a mom to our kids at the orphanage.

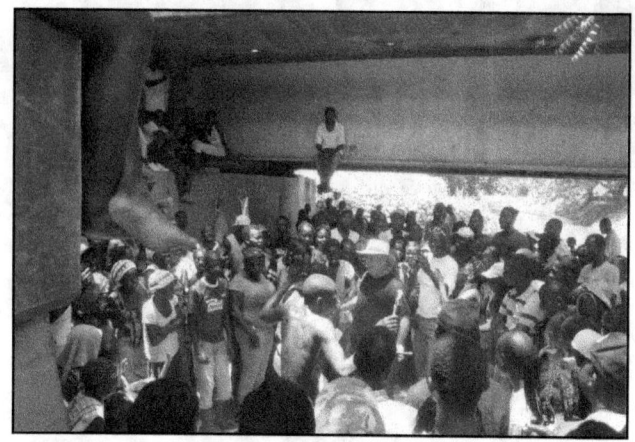

A VooDoo religious service 2011.

CHAPTER 12

Mission Trip to Dominican Republic and Haiti, October 2008

It is a man's sympathy with all creatures that truly makes him a man. Until he extends his circle of compassion to all living things, man himself will not find peace.

—ALBERT SCHWEITZER

Our mission trip to Haiti in October 2008 included fifty chiropractors and fifty chiropractic assistants, who cared for more than 56,000 people in four days.

To prepare to see thousands of patients in the world's poorest countries, Todd and I had to lead by example. We had to clear our minds of everything but chiropractic. We had got together four days before the mission at Camp David, a retreat high atop the mountains overlooking the city of Santiago in Dominican Republic. It has spectacular views, and the location serves as a training site for the leaders of our chiropractic mission teams.

We spent two days in pure chiropractic thought before beginning the tremendous project of coordinating the lectures and education we were giving to the medical directors of several hospitals throughout the country. Dr. Pat Gentempo and I, along with JC and Dr. Aura, educated the staff and medical directors of the Caribbean's most prestigious hospital, Holmes Medical Center of Santiago.

Dr. Gentempo and I spent hours explaining the science, philosophy, and art of chiropractic. Meanwhile, Todd worked with Sor Teodora to assemble, schedule, and transport the chiropractic teams to their destinations. Each team consisted of a chiropractor, a chiropractic student, and a mission guide, and were sent to churches, orphanages, schools, nursing homes, and even jails. Teams were sent to the ghettos, mountaintop villages, farms, and cities throughout the country.

In preparation for my voyage to Haiti, I wanted to climb the highest peak in the Caribbean, Pico Duarte, and spend two days in chiropractic meditation. Early in the morning of September 23, 2008, I landed in Santiago, rented a car, and headed, chiropractic table in hand, to Pico Duarte. A few hours later, I arrived in a beautiful city that lies below this majestic mountain.

Arribicoa is lush with tropical plants, fruits, and palm trees. I immediately drove to the city's central police station. With my table in hand and my mission mindset, I walked into the station and opened my table, then proceeded to adjust every police officer and employee. Policemen were handing their shotguns to other officers as their turn on my table approached. Others were on the phone calling friends, family, and other officers to come to the station as soon as possible. After I adjusted seventy or eighty people, a group of policeman took me out to lunch. Of course, we ate the best chicken, rice, and beans, and a strong brew of Dominican coffee launched me on my way.

I set up my table in the center of the city and adjusted two hundred people over the next four or five hours. I know that sounds like a lot of people, but in these impoverished countries, people just line up and look forward to getting on the table. God guided my hands to areas that needed adjusting. Full spine diversified takes less than a minute for an adjustment, and the citizens of poor countries are very easy to adjust because very few of them are overweight. Audibles are common in people over ninety.

I found a charming hotel three-quarters of the way up Pico Duarte. For forty dollars a night, I had a delightful cabin with a kitchen, living room, den, and balcony overlooking the valley below. The next day I arose early and was hiking through the trails above the hotel when I came upon a lovely old church. I sat in front of the church, gazing at the city that was enveloped in the mountains below. A slight drizzle was moistening my pages of *The Chiropractor* during my daily reading. I was drafting my spiritual chiropractic talk that I would be presenting to the many students, chiropractors, pastors, and laypeople who I would be speaking to during our chiropractic mission. As I contemplated the vastness and power of the universe and pondered the writings of D.D. Palmer, an enormous rainbow emerged. It started close to where I was sitting and went across the entire valley. It lasted for more than two hours.

I voyaged over the mountaintops of Pico Duarte and came upon a magical city. The climate was completely different than in any other part of the country. It was a cool 65 degrees with a rich blue sky. I was told by the locals that it is like this here in Constanza every day. The city was in the midst of their yearly festival—an ideal time to start adjusting. I set up my table in a square that was blocked off for the night's festivities, and adjusted three hundred people in six hours. I then took several hours off to eat with a wonderful family at their small abode. They were very appreciative of my adjustments to their grandma and infant child. Grandma made a marvelous home-cooked Dominican meal: rice, chicken, and beans followed by the world's best cup of coffee.

Nightfall approached, and I was back at the festival. Anthony Santos was playing, and I was adjusting. Omega was next, and I was still adjusting. Anthony Santos (bachata) and Omega (merengue) are two of the most popular Dominican musical groups. I finished adjusting at one in the morning.

I arrived at Camp David early Tuesday morning. Todd scheduled a chiropractic and spiritual hike through the mountains, and JC, Aura, and Genopolis, life students John Palmer, Jason Brown, Danielle Drobbin, Dina, and I followed Todd's instructions to a T. We were rewarded with the most inspiring chiropractic hike imaginable.

A few hours later John Palmer, Jason Brown, and I departed for the world's most impoverished land, Haiti. I had been driving for about three hours when we noticed that the terrain was changing dramatically. We were met at the border by Hughes Bastian. As we crossed over the bridge to Haiti, I gazed down below and noticed hundreds of people in the river. People were washing their bodies as well as their clothes.

As we entered Haiti, our senses were immediately heightened. There was no vegetation, garbage was everywhere, and our noses were struck by a terrible odor. In 1925, Haiti was lush, with 60 percent of its original forest covering the lands and mountainous regions. Since then, the population has cut down all but an estimated 2 percent of its original forest cover, and in the process has destroyed fertile farmland soils. All we could see was dirt for miles. We were told that erosion was severe in the mountainous areas.

Most Haitian logging is done to produce charcoal, the country's chief source of fuel. The plight of Haiti's forests has attracted international attention and has led to numerous reforestation efforts, but they have met with little success. Needless to say, Haiti was in an environmental crisis when we were there.

Chiropractic mission work is certainly not boring. We were on a mission from God and D.D. Palmer. We arrived at a hospital, and hundreds of people were waiting for us on three separate floors. I adjusted about 350 people in five hours. Two life students utilized motion palpation and prepared each patient for my adjustment. People of all ages and conditions mounted my portable chiropractic tables. Many had great difficulty but were helped by two of our assistants.

Most people in Haiti only speak French and Creole, so I had a translator write a sign for me that said "Nice to meet you. Face up. Face down. On your side." I would just point to the sign indicating how I wanted them on the table.

Many patients had serious problems. People presented with oozing tumors and giant goiters. They were promptly adjusted and referred to the two medical doctors who were working downstairs. For their medical visits, the patients had to pay a dollar. Most did not have the dollar and had to wait until mission doctors arrived.

Most patients had neuromusculoskeletal symptoms and protein deficiencies. Some had diphtheria, croup, inflammation of the bowels, or pneumonia. Many of the patients responded well with one or two treatments.

The chronic diseases would take from two weeks to two months to affect a permanent cure.

The sun goes down at six o'clock, and since there was no electricity in the whole country, most people went to sleep around seven. I did find a candlelit restaurant and candlelit discothèque. It was exhilarating to walk through the candlelit streets. My two students were a little nervous as we walked into the butane lamp-light club. All we could see was bright white eyes and incandescent teeth. The good news was that beer was only twenty-five cents a bottle. A few rounds for the life students and me only set me back three dollars, including a generous tip. We had a late night out and were home sleeping by ten o'clock.

I was awakened at four thirty in the morning by the loudest, most obnoxious squealing noise I had ever heard. A pig was being slaughtered for the next day's meals. Now I understood why I was given ear plugs when we arrived. At five o'clock the church bells rung, and thousands of people were going to the Catholic church or the Baptist church in full daylight.

We were scheduled to see patients from seven in the morning to six in the evening, with a small break for lunch. Breakfast ran late, and we arrived at seven fifteen to hundreds of people. All three floors were filled with people waiting for us. By eleven, the two students were fading fast. John Palmer had to take a few hours off since his stomach was off. When he returned, Jason Brown almost collapsed. He ran off to take a nap, but diarrhea had struck.

I adjusted an astronomical number of people, all the way through to the end. Three tables were set for me, and I just moved in a circle from table to table. Translators helped the people on and off the tables. Three days and a thousand adjustments later, we were on our way back to Dominican Republic, where we would be joining our colleagues at an all-inclusive resort in the tropical paradise of Puerta Plata.

I was thinking as we are driving how nice it was going to be to take a hot shower and feel some air conditioning once again. After all, it was a brutal 101 degrees for three straight days, and all of the showers were cold and without water pressure. I was suddenly surprised, amazed, and astonished by the sight I witnessing out of our car window. There were fifty or more people gathered together in a small area made out of concrete. Out of the fifty is a line of about ten more people. At the end of the line, a person was pumping water out of a well into a bucket. The buckets were being passed down the line, and a few people stood atop chairs and were throwing the water on the heads of the crowd. Others were pouring soap solutions, and yet others were scrubbing using archaic brushes. Imagine taking a shower fifty people deep. Imagine no running water, and that an outhouse is a luxury. I needed to stop and take a minute to thank God for my three days of cold water with bad pressure.

We arrived in Dominican Republic to serve chiropractic. First we had the opportunity to spend some quality time in a chiropractic seminar at the all-inclusive beach resort. It felt like paradise. During the days that followed, we served thousands of Dominican people our gift of chiropractic.

After the mission trip, Dr. Matthew J. Haumesser sent me this a letter:

> It has been a couple weeks, and I have had some time to reflect on the entire experience. I hope that the people of Dominican Republic got a fraction of what I feel like I have received from the Chiromissions trip. I now have a new perspective on gratitude and what is truly important. There were three things that had a profound impact on me, and I would like to share them with you.
>
> 1: On the first full day of mission work, I got to see the power of one adjustment. I saw how one adjustment can change not just the life of one person but the entire community. A student and I adjusted a woman who had nothing—no food, no water, no clothes. She had walked by earlier, and we were trying to get her to come get adjusted. She wouldn't make eye contact, let alone come over. Some of the taxi drivers who were lingering around told us not to bother, that she was crazy and that no one deals with her at all. After an hour or so, she walked back through and sat on a curb fifty yards away. We walked over and convinced her to allow us to adjust her. After that, we saw someone come out and give her some food and milk. We could see that they

saw her in different light after we adjusted her (or turned her light back on). Also, my student gave her a shirt to wear.

2. On the last full day, I went to Villa Progresso. Here I met an eleven-year-old boy who took a liking to me. He walked me around the village so I could adjust all of his family, friends, and neighbors. He was awesome. If I was going too slow, he would say, "Vamos, Mateo." Let's go, Matt. I had given him ten pesos for helping me. After an hour or so he said he was thirsty, so we walked to a store. He asked if I was thirsty. I said yes and told him I would buy us some drinks. He ran ahead and spent the ten pesos on a drink for me and him. That hit me hard. Here was a kid who had nothing, and he spent his only ten pesos on me. Talk about the true meaning of giving. I later gave him 150 pesos, and you would have thought I had given him a solid gold brick.

3. Before my flight out, I was killing time until it was time to head home. I had you adjust me, Peter, and I was so honored to be able to adjust you. That, too, was huge. So, Doc, thanks. I hope in some way I have helped the wonderful people of the DR. I know they and all of you have changed me. I will be back. I don't know when, but I will be back. I plan on bringing my wife and maybe two chiropractor friends of mine.

Much thanks,
Dr. Matthew J. Haumesser

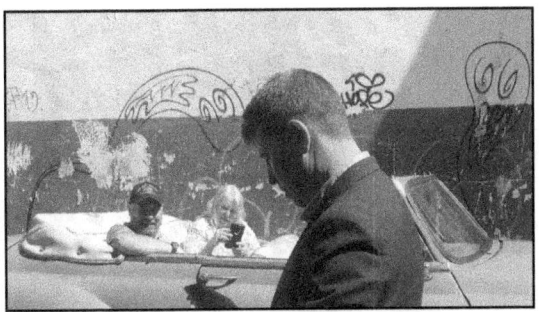

Havana, Cuba currently has a cell phone signal.

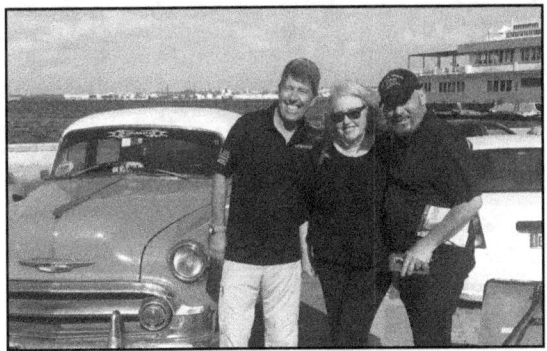

Brad Rauch, DC; Ellen Coyne, DC and I in Havana, Cuba. We are planning a future mission trip to Cuba.

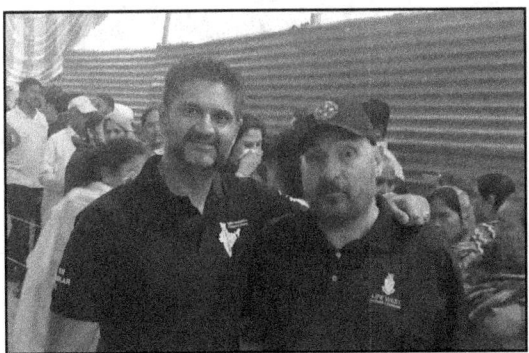

Jimmy Nanda, DC and I on a mission trip to India. Jimmy is the Chairman of the Board at Life West Chiropractic College.

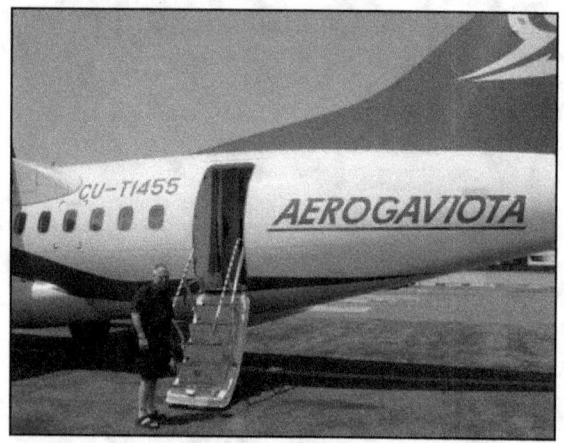

Our plane to cuba.

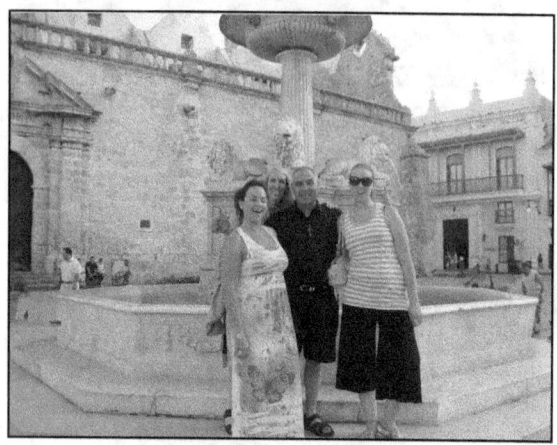

Downtown Old Havana, Cuba 2009

CHAPTER 13

Mission Trip to Cuba, January 2009

Many believe that self-help and self-improvement is about rags to riches, failure to success, and so forth, when indeed it is the beginning of a journey into self-discovery. Inside every human being is an eternal truth and a life purpose. Using our mind power is simply starting the engine on that journey of self-discovery and highest self-actualization.

—ELDON TAYLOR

In January 2009 Mission Life International sent a chiropractic mission team of ten chiropractors, three chiropractic students, three chiropractic assistants, and 1onechiropractic office manager to bring chiropractic and humanitarian supplies to the people of Cuba. It was the first time an organized chiropractic mission trip actually made it to Cuba. I led the five-day mission trip to the communist nation at a time when new hope had emerged among the Cuban residents. In return, the group made new friendships and brought home a better understanding of the plight of people on the island.

Dr. Joseph Cucci and I had gone early to set up the Haiti-Dominican Republic chiropractic mission trip. We rented two homes in Port au Prince, Haiti, and met with several pastors and medical professionals. We hired professional photographers, a video crew, and jeeps for the chiropractic trek from one end of Haiti, through the middle of the country, and finally to Dominican Republic. We were planning to see patients in churches, village centers, and hospitals, and we knew that people were going to be waiting in line for days to get adjusted.

We stayed in the DR for two days and then drove sixteen hours to Haiti and back. We made our arrangements and flew to Nassau, Bahamas. In Nassau we met the rest of our Cuban mission team, seventeen people from California, Delaware, Indiana, Illinois, Minnesota, North Dakota, New York, New Jersey, New Hampshire, and Pennsylvania. The next day we boarded an old Russian small-propeller plane. We encountered turbulence for the entire hour-long ride.

We touched down in Havana and were greeted by hundreds of Cuban workers wearing swine flu masks. It was really eerie, as was going through an extensive and enduring customs protocol. We finally exited the airport.

We felt as if we had gone back in time. Most of the cars were made in the 1950s, and they all ran and looked as if they were brand new. One of our taxis was a 1957 Chevy station wagon that could easily hold ten. We stayed in a beautiful hotel that overlooked Havana's majestic harbor. The entrance to the harbor was guarded by a four-hundred-year-old fort. The Spanish had raised this fort next to the harbor entrance between 1589 and 1630, with the objective of warding off attacks by pirates and enemy fleets. In 1845 a huge lighthouse was built adjacent to the fort, making the entrance to Havana even more picturesque.

The architecture was stupendous, giving Havana an appearance of Spain, the Caribbean, and Italy mixed together. There were statues and fountains in the spacious old squares. We encountered many old forts and heavenly churches. We visited appetizing restaurants with musicians serenading us as we enjoyed one delicious meal after the next.

The highlight of the evening was when we witnessed soldiers dressed in the uniforms of the British redcoats performing a curfew time firing of the cannon, as the British had when they captured Havana back in 1762. It was a ceremony of sound and lights performed on the ramparts with great fanfare. It was a great favorite with tourists and Cuban children, who were brought in from the countryside as a treat during the holidays.

The following day we set out on our chiropractic mission work. We boarded a ferry that took us across the harbor to Regla, where the common folk lived. It was completely different from the downtown tourist area of Old Havana, where we were staying. As we walked by old, worn-out buildings and shacks, we caught glimpses of life through wide-open front doors. In nearly every house there was a vase bulging with fresh wildflowers placed in the most obvious location on the table or counter. The beauty of God's creation set among these shacks of poverty was strange to see—not the flowers, but the wonderful Cuban people. There are no clocks, no alarms, no rushing; just the rising sun and the clip-clop-tick-tock of horses' hooves set the pace for these folks.

We set off to a converted house/church, where we were scheduled to begin at nine o'clock. We arrived to a multitude of Cuban patients, who had put on their best clothes. It didn't matter to the kids that some of them didn't have shoes or that a shirt was buttoned all wrong. They jockeyed for position to get a glimpse of us. Not too close, just close enough. These were simple, honest, and hardworking people who had waited patiently to see the chiropractors from the United States. We addressed a large crowd that had assembled in the church, telling them the chiropractic story. We then set up our adjusting rooms. We were not allowed to bring portable chiropractic tables into Cuba, but our hosts had made a number of fantastic tables for us to use. They were set up in several rooms.

I was surprised and encouraged to see how much Cubans can do with so little; it was truly a testament to the world that the mighty hand of God was upon them. The poverty was devastating, as was the customer service offered in all public places. In spite of this, the Cuban church where we were stationed was growing more and more every day. About 90 percent of the church population was between the ages of thirteen and thirty.

While we were adjusting, we saw the thirst, enthusiasm, and desire the Cubans had to learn more about chiropractic. The beautiful things they did with little or no resources at all deeply ministered to our spirits.

The next day part of our team went about an hour outside of Havana to the countryside. We set up our adjusting rooms in a small church and the attached house. As we walked around, we noticed that comfort was a foreign concept. Many of the Cubans living in the home had severe disabilities. The beds were simple slabs of wood, many without a pillow or even a cover. The pastor had made the floors himself to make more room for the people who lived there.

Whenever we broke for lunch or dinner, we were told that honored guests eat first, everyone else later. They had so little, yet what they had was offered as completely ours. They gave what they had from the heart. Someone commented that they liked the small, old-fashioned coffee machine, and they wanted to give it to her.

The kitchen and eating area floor was plain concrete but was swept and mopped perfectly clean. Life was simple. Life was slow. Generations had been born right on this property, and shacks had been added to accommodate marriages. The family worked hard to live; it showed in the roughness of their feet, hands, and faces, but their hearts were as warm and innocent as a child's.

All the children in the little community were drawn to us, and we felt like pied pipers. Everywhere we went, eight or nine children would follow us. The digital camera always brought fun, laughter, and smiles, as it would inspire the children to transform themselves into athletes, circus artists, clowns, and acrobats. They would start posing for the camera and do gravity-defying cartwheels and flips, then immediately want to see their pictures. Their smiles and laughter were like a penetrating dagger headed straight to the heart. They couldn't stop their tongues once their hearts were given. I guess no one had told them they were dreadfully poor. All they cared about was a quick game of soccer, which they played with a ball made out of some rubber that they picked up in a garbage dump. Some kids rode their rickety old bicycles with flat tires and bent wheels. Did they know their clothes were tattered? Did they know their homes were shacks?

As we left in the car, the kids ran alongside, waving a hundred times. With each wave they looked us in the eye, and the last wave meant as much as the first. If you are not willing to give your heart away, you should never come to Cuba.

One of the mission team chiropractors related the following story to me.

What an incredible experience I had in Cuba. It was five of the most meaningful days of my life. We spent weeks training, preparing, and praying for God to use our seventeen-person team as He saw fit. We went to be a blessing to the wonderful people of Cuba, but we were blessed far more. We had the privilege of adjusting in homes and sharing chiropractic in churches. We built relationships with the many beautiful Cuban people and delivered pure chiropractic with God's love to as many people as possible.

We were humbled to see many chiropractic miracles while we were there. We saw God working through us as we taught and adjusted in Havana and Regla. We heard great life-changing testimonies from those whom we had adjusted the day before. Although we adjusted our brothers and sisters in Cuba, our team was also ministered to from our Cuban brothers through their dedication and love of God. We saw God work despite the very limited resources and the many hardships that must be endured to carry out God's mission in Cuba. Speaking for our team and myself, this chiropractic mission trip was a life-changing experience for both our brothers in Cuba and us.

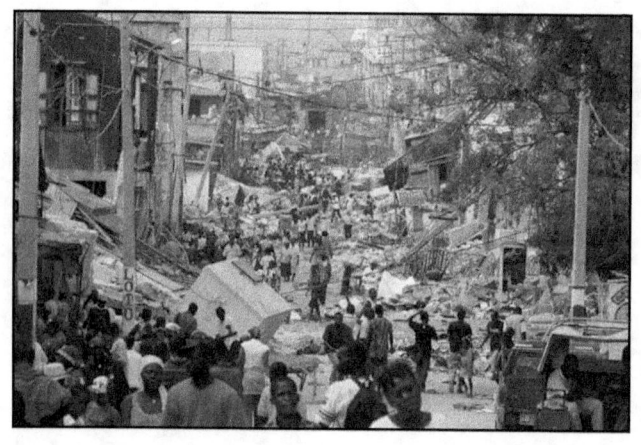

Port Au Prince, Haiti days after the earthquake. January 2010

CHAPTER 14

Haiti Earthquake 2010

The ability to change your life comes from the power of love in your heart. Love connects you to other people's emotions. It's the ultimate source of emotional fuel, so plug into it!

—PEGGY MCCOLL

The island of Hispaniola comprises the two countries of Haiti and Dominican Republic, with Haiti to the west and Dominican Republic to the east. The two countries couldn't be more different, with Dominican Republic enjoying a booming tourism industry, and Haiti struggling as one of the poorest countries in the world.

On January 12, 2010, at 3:45 in the afternoon—less than twenty-four hours after I had left—a massive 7.1 earthquake struck Haiti about ten miles outside of the capital of Port-au-Prince. More than 300,000 people were killed, and 2.3 million were left homeless and without clean water or food. It was perhaps the worst earthquake in modern history.

Our chiropractic mission tour that month had begun on January 2, 2010, in Dominican Republic. Our mission team, twenty people strong, spent five days serving in that country, and then on January 7, 2010, we entered into Haiti. We ministered in the town of Ouanaminthe until January 10, 2010. The mission trip concluded, and most of our team returned to the United States that same day. Some went back to Dominican Republic for a few days of rest and relaxation at the awesome Dominican beaches. I went on to Port-au-Prince to visit some friends who were once patients at my New York chiropractic office. I left Port-au-Prince the next day to return back to my home and family in New York. The earthquake struck the next day.

God spoke to me on that day. All I could think about was returning to Haiti as soon as possible to help in any way I could. I phoned Saurel Charles, a New York taxi driver who was once a famous actor in Haiti. His stage name had been Boss Massel. Boss had been a regular patient at my chiropractic office in New York City for a number of years, and he owned a large piece of property in Port-au-Prince.

"Boss, how are you?" I asked, "Doc, my homeland has been destroyed. Family members are missing. I can't get through. Phone lines are down. I don't have any money. Can you buy me a plane ticket?"

"I'll buy two," I answered. "We leave for Dominican Republic tomorrow. The Port-au-Prince airport has been destroyed. We'll have to drive from Santo Domingo, in the DR, to Port-au-Prince." My wife and three kids were hysterical. They did not want me to go. CNN was showing live footage of the devastation, and more earthquakes were happening. But God had spoken—I must go. I sent out an email to thirty thousand people; I needed a team to come down to Haiti for a rescue effort.

Boss and I arrived in Santo Domingo on January 15. We drove six hours, and just short of three days after the massive earthquake, we arrived in Port-au-Prince. It was a living hell. Death was everywhere, and thousands of people were crying. Boss Massel's house miraculously withstood the shaking, and most of his family was safe. However, some of his cousins and many friends were gone. We searched and searched and searched for survivors. Some were found buried under the earth; some were never found. We took in many children to Boss's house.

We assessed the situation for our most immediate and important essentials—we needed tents and food—and I left Port-au-Prince on January 18 to return to New York to acquire our necessities. I was there for a short two-day stay with my family and just enough time to get my chiropractic practice in order.

I quickly had a team of ten chiropractors and seven Christian missionaries ready to go to Haiti and serve. My friend and colleague Brad Rauch, DC, raised

$50,000, and twenty-five water filtration systems were delivered to my office. I returned to Haiti with my new team on January 20, just eight days after the earthquake.

On the flight back to Haiti, I video-interviewed every passenger on the JetBlue airplane. Most of them were doctors going to serve in hospitals and perform surgeries. One of the people I interviewed was the president of the Lions Clubs International. He informed me that the Lions were sending two thousand tents to Haiti. Fifty of those tents were now designated for our mission.

Once we arrived in Santo Domingo, we rented four large SUVs and filled them with food and water. We drove through the night and arrived in Port-au-Prince the next morning.

We had multiple objectives when we started the mission. We wanted to offer chiropractic care to the people, whether injured or not; bring state-of-the-art water filtration systems to communities; distribute food and water; and offer hope, faith, and service to humanity. We hauled around our portable tables to wherever chiropractic was needed, installed ten water filtration systems in ten different locations, and ministered to the traumatized and bereaved.

Every day for the next two weeks we ventured into the fields behind the US Embassy, where we offered low-tech bandaging and wound care. We brought our chiropractic tables into the makeshift tent cities around the corner from the Capitol building. We checked and adjusted thousands of people. Two our team associates served in the hospitals, assisting in amputations and delivering babies.

As we worked on these people, they told us that they had not had a drink of water in six days. "*We need food and water!*" We provided food, water, and adjustments throughout the city. As we drove around the city providing water to the thirsty, we noticed that there were no other groups providing this service.

The water systems we set up provided clean drinking water to entire communities. Among the recipients was a makeshift hospital in the rubble of the worst-hit section in the city, a community ambulance service that was nearly totally destroyed, the house of the pastor whose community we adopted, Boss's home, and a community church associated with Stepping Stones Ministry. We also distributed our water filtration systems to hospitals, fire houses, and police stations.

By coincidence, our Stepping Stones Ministry building and safe haven was in the same neighborhood where Boss owned his property. The community was almost completely destroyed. The school, church, and most of the homes were gone. Luckily, the Stepping Stones Ministry lost only part of their building. We decided to adopt the community. The fifty tents donated to Mission Life International by the Lions Clubs International finally arrived and were assembled on Boss's property.

One day I interviewed a popular Haitian musician, who told me that he sat down with his band to practice every day at 3:30. His current band employed his three kids. Moments before beginning their practice rehearsal on January 12, he and his kids were visiting family across the street and enjoying a delicious barbeque roast. The band left the picnic, headed home to rehearse, and sat down with their instruments.

Suddenly, the ground began to shake. Everyone stood up and tried to hold on to the walls. The earth trembled for forty-five seconds, and then the building that they had occupied only moments before came crashing down into their building. All of their family and friends at the barbeque perished underneath the rubble. The musician's neighbor, a medical doctor, grabbed him, and the next thing he remembered was assisting in amputations. The musician recounted, "If your arm or your leg were stuck in the rubble, you could die unless it was surgically removed." He helped the doctor with amputations for several weeks.

Brad Rauch, my colleague who raised $50,000, and I were exhausted from days of non-stop relief work. We were sleeping inside Boss Massel's house on January 21 when woke up to an underground eruption—a 6.1 aftershock had struck. The ground was trembling as concrete fell. Brad and I ran outside to find our team safe and sound in our jeeps and vans. The next day we experienced more aftershocks.

We ran more than twenty mission trips and brought over four hundred chiropractors to Haiti in the next two years.

When thousands of displaced families are living together in overcrowded and unhygienic tent cities, outbreaks of cholera are common, so it was no surprise when there was a serious outbreak in the area. People were now afraid to come on our mission trips. I held strong; I knew we needed to be adjusting people with cholera and checking their spines. More chiropractic missionaries finally came down to work with us.

I have a profound love for the people of Haiti, and I will never forget the devastation that the earthquake of 2010 wreaked on the country and its people. I have since taken hundreds people on mission trips to this impoverished land, but there is much to be done, even ten years later.

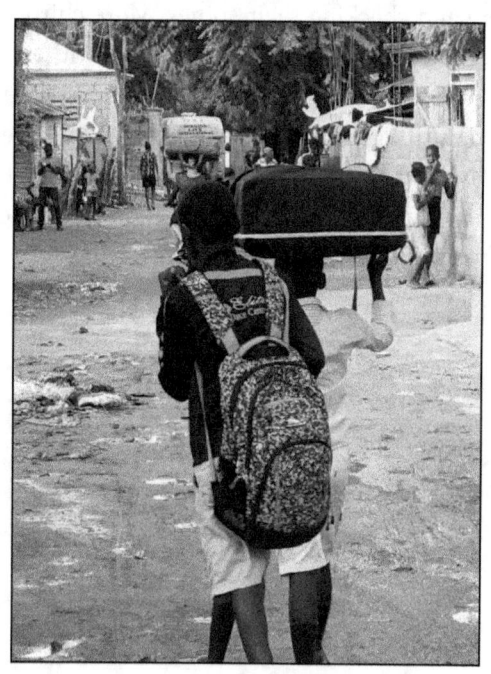

Children from our orphanage
carrying our tables. 2018

CHAPTER 15

One Year after the Earthquake

You have got to discover you, what you do, and trust it.

—BARBRA STREISAND

One year after the enormous earthquake in Haiti, the people were still suffering tremendously. The earthquake had compounded pre-existing issues of structural problems, severe poverty, low development, and limited access to education, health, and sanitation services.

Many of our team members experienced digestive disturbances after drinking bottled water, and our digestive systems were getting back to normal a year later. I experienced nightmares during my first week back in the States and still experienced nightmares, but only every once in a while. They weren't bad after a year, but they were in the beginning.

In the year following the earthquake, we returned to Port au Prince ten times with ten teams of chiropractors and missionaries. In that time, we raised thousands of dollars for food and opened a free chiropractic clinic and an orphanage. I also teamed up with four other chiropractors to open two chiropractic offices in Dominican Republic. During this same time I was appointed by the World Chiropractic Alliance as its non-governmental organization (NGO) representative to the United Nations' Department of Public Information.

A colleague and I attended a briefing at the United Nations, DPI/NGO Relations Cluster entitled "Disaster Relief and Preparedness: Haiti, A Year Later." The four panelists reported that one year after the earthquake, United Nations relief work was still ongoing. They said that the UN had provided water to 8 million people per day, food to 2 million per month, and 31,000 transitional shelters. They had provided housing, education, water, and health care, and created 250,000 jobs. They had three pilot programs underway for fourteen new neighborhoods in Port au Prince. Between February and November 2010, 240,000 people were employed through cash- and food-for-work schemes through 231 projects. The World Food Program reached 400,000 beneficiaries through similar programs, which focused on employing people for rubble clearance and canal cleaning. Many thousands of teachers and education staff were trained, including in psychosocial support for traumatized children. Hundreds of thousands of school children benefited from provisions of basic learning materials. Almost three thousand temporary learning spaces replaced destroyed schools, and 1.1 million children received daily meals through the National School Feeding Programme. By May 2010, 900,000 vaccinations were administered to vulnerable populations, and 345,000 health kits with medicines and supplies such as antibiotics, vaccines, anesthetics, and analgesics were distributed.

After the presentation, we were allowed to ask the panelists questions. I needed to be diplomatic even though I was raging inside, as it was my first day as a chiropractic representative to the UN. I had not seen any evidence of the food or water distribution, and I certainly had not seen 31,000 shelters. I had not heard of any jobs for the Haitian people. Perhaps foreigners were getting the 240,000 jobs. The kids we saw were going to schools in churches, and the teachers were not being paid. None of the teachers we knew in Port au Prince knew anything about the educational materials being distributed.

I said to the panelists, "Thank you for all the work that you have been doing in Haiti and for spending time with us today. I am a chiropractor, and I represent the World Chiropractic Alliance. I was in Haiti the day before the earthquake, and I have returned ten times in the year since. I have many friends who are in Port au Prince. My friends do not know where the water distribution is, they do not know where the food distribution is, and they do not know anything about the transitional housing and fourteen new communities being developed. My friends would like to have paying jobs. Would you be so kind as to give me the lists of these sites so that I can pass them on to my friends?"

Can you guess what the answer was? "We don't have those lists. You need to call UNICEF." I later called UNICEF and never did see any of those lists. I learned that the response activities of UN and partners for 2010 required $1.5 billion. Not one of my friends in Port au Prince saw any of this money

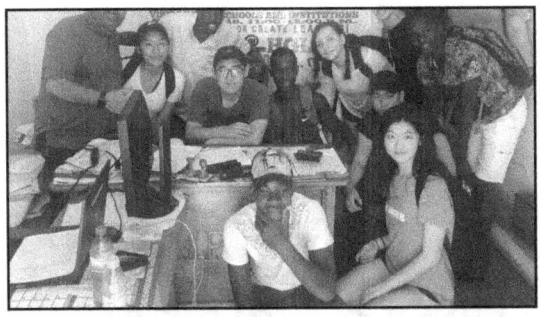

Every January I take a group of high school students from Europe, Asia and Australia to Haiti.

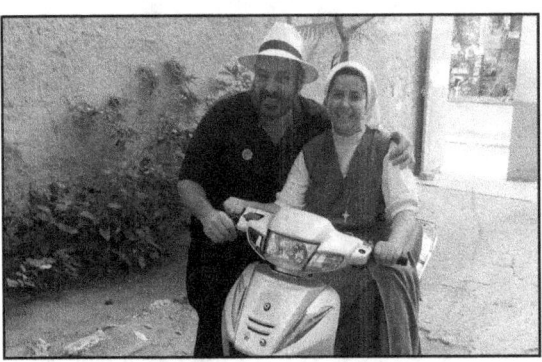

Sor Alexandre is a catholic nun from Colombia and has been serving in Haiti for over 10 years. She reminds me of Sally Fields in the flying nun.

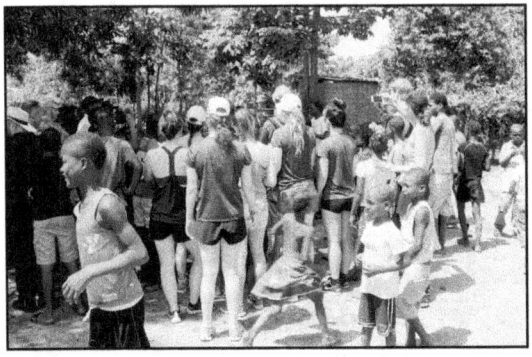

Chiropractic generates a lot of excitement.

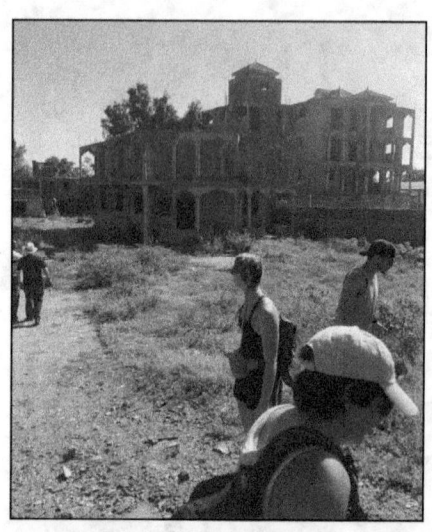

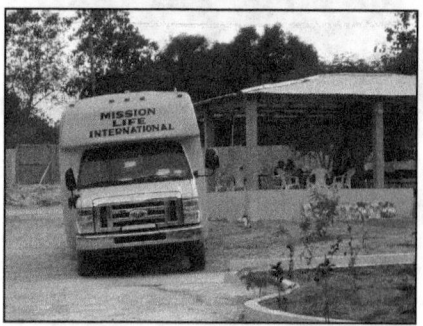

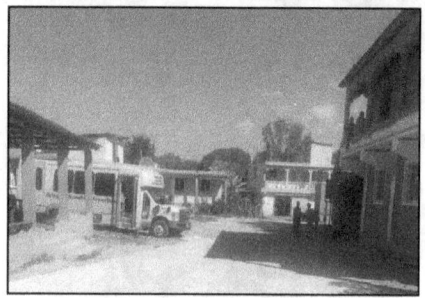

Our property in Ouanaminthe, Haiti in 2016 and then again in 2019.

CHAPTER 16

Mission Trip to Haiti and Dominican Republic, February 2012

In February 2012 Mission Life International moved all of its assets to Ouanaminthe, Haiti. Ouanaminthe is a small city on the border with Dominican Republic. It was going to be a much easier location to work in because of its vicinity to Dominican Republic. It is also close to three international airports. The airport in Port au Prince was destroyed during the earthquake, and travel had become very difficult.

We had plans to house fifty-nine children in one home and twenty-nine children in another home. Mission Life International had rehabilitated water and sanitation systems at health clinics and youth centers and helped build latrines, showers, and safe water points in the capital, and now we were going to do the same for Ouanaminthe, Fort Liberte, and Malfiti. We had trained volunteers, and we educated people on good health and disease-prevention practices, such as effective handwashing and hygienic food preparation.

On my third mission trip to Dominican Republic that year, we had a team of eighteen chiropractors and thirty chiropractic students serving love and chiropractic to the poorer areas of Dominican Republic. Part of our team also visited Haiti.

We were able to visit with our guide, Eddie, who had been on all twenty-two of our post-earthquake Haiti mission trips. Eddie had served chiropractic with his heart and soul. He translated for all of our teams and told the chiropractic story to thousands of people. He protected us from harm and wanted to go to chiropractic school. He was already fluent in the chiropractic philosophy. On our second trip to Haiti, I had given him a number of chiropractic books, and he has mastered them all. Eddie absorbed everything chiropractic. He told a group of chiropractors on one of our missions that he thought Jesus was the first chiropractor. After all, he had seen many chiropractic miracles in those two short years. He knew as much about chiropractic as chiropractors who have been in practice for ten years.

While we were talking, Eddie said that he had witnessed the nearly 25,000 children who suffered from severe acute malnutrition. Many were dying daily. One in three children in Haiti was estimated to be chronically malnourished. I had seen for myself that people who were living in the tent cities needed to be protected from harm, including sexual violence. The major needs for affected populations were sanitation, waste management, and drinking water, especially for those in the tent cities. Another worry was the cholera. Over three thousand people died from cholera because of the unsanitary conditions and the state of the water.

One night I was driving by myself on a desolate road on my way from Santiago, Dominican Republic, to Ouanaminthe, Haiti, on my way to deliver toothbrushes, toothpaste, soap, and shampoo to our Haitian orphanages. I was also finding housing for the ten chiropractic missionaries who would be arriving in a few days. I planned to stay the night at a friend's house in a border town called Dajabon in Dominican Republic. I had driven this road many times, mostly during the day. As I got closer and closer to Haiti, the terrain changed dramatically, going from a fertile and lush landscape to desert. Dominican Republic has beautiful waterfalls, spectacular beaches, and flower-filled landscape and fresh fruits and vegetables everywhere.

When I crossed the small, overcrowded bridge to enter Haiti during the daytime, I would immediately encounter thousands of beggars, huge flies and mosquitoes, large pigs, and garbage everywhere. There was no electricity in most of Haiti, so the people cut down the trees to make charcoal for cooking and lighting, making the oxygen-carbon dioxide balance askew. Since the soil was infertile, the Haitians had to go to

Dominican Republic to buy fruits and vegetables. Most people couldn't afford diapers, and children defecated on the side of the road. What a mess.

Baboom!!! I heard a huge backfire, and suddenly my 4-wheel drive vehicle stalled and shut down. I called the owner of my borrowed car, but he must have been sleeping.

Innate told me that the jeep was out of gas. I waved down the lone motorcycle that passed by fifteen minutes later. He drove me to a friend's house, and his friend siphoned gas into a container. Ninety minutes later, we arrived back at the jeep. The car still wouldn't start. The owner finally awoke and told me that the jeep had run out of propane and that I should just hit a switch under the dashboard to change the fuel to gasoline. Who knew that the car had a propane tank in the trunk? It turned out that many people used propane to fuel their cars in the DR and Haiti.

The next day I crossed the border and entered Haiti. Nothing had changed since the earthquake two years before. Actually, things had worsened—a cholera outbreak had occurred. I had adjusted many with cholera. At the orphanage, all of the more than one hundred children had fungal infections on their heads. Some of the children were younger than two years old and were awaiting their first toothbrush. Pastors from many churches were at the orphanage and gathered round to wait to be adjusted. They asked for me to bring back a message to my church in New York City: *Please help us.*

Please do not forget us. Please adopt our churches here in Haiti and make us part of your church in New York.

The rest of our chiropractic mission team arrived. We were staying at homes with outhouses for bathrooms, no showers, no air conditioning, and water that we cannot even touch. We could only drink small bottled waters. Showers were buckets of bottled water with brown soap. We adjusted thousands of kids while we were in Haiti, and in several hospitals we adjusted all the medical doctors, nurses, and patients, and we even checked and adjusted newborns. We adjusted thousands of people in tent cities and nursing homes.

It was an incredible mission trip. It was great to have a new beginning in Ouanaminthe. We had not served there since January 2010. I reunited with many Haitian people who had become like family to me. They really needed our help in this part of Haiti. There was no electricity in this small city, no running water, hospitals without X-ray machines, and people were living in mud huts. Aluminum roofs were a luxury. The people were poor, but they were the most wonderful people I had ever met.

After our chiropractic mission trip in Haiti was over, we drove to Puerto Plata, Dominican Republic. This was my favorite part of our Hispaniola Chiropractic Mission Trip. On each trip from Haiti to Dominican Republic I was reminded of the famous literary work of Dante Alighieri. While I was living and studying in an Italian monastery in 1980, I had to read *The*

Divine Comedy, Dante's epic poem completed in 1320. It is widely considered the preeminent work of Italian literature, and is seen as one of the greatest works of world literature. The poem's imaginative and allegorical vision of the afterlife is a culmination of the medieval worldview as it had developed in the Western church. It is divided into three parts: "The Inferno," "Purgatorio," and "Paradiso." On the surface, the poem describes Dante's travels through Hell, Purgatory, and Heaven, but at a deeper level, it allegorically represents the soul's journey toward God.

I couldn't help but to think that in many ways this mission that I was journeying on was the Divine Comedy. The island of Hispaniola was made up of the Inferno. Many areas in Haiti were a living hell, especially for those people so poor that their children were literally dying from starvation, who were sick and disabled and didn't have any healthcare, who were living in tent cities, and who had gangrenous extremities waiting for their amputations.

Purgatory was in the border towns. These Haitian towns had some form of income. They bought products in Dominican Republic and sold them to Haitian people in towns farther away from the border. Dominican Republic would open its borders on Mondays and Fridays so that the Haitians could come and purchase products that they could then sell.

Paradise. Paradiso. This was the rich culture of Dominican Republic and home of the happiest people in the world, people who were forever dancing, who presented us with huge hugs and eye-beaming love after each chiropractic adjustment. The gorgeous mountains and lush beaches of Dominican Republic—paradise. Yes, it was paradise for the tourists and most Dominicans but purgatory for many Haitians in Dominican-Haitian villages. These were Haitians who had left Haiti and entered Dominican Republic illegally. Even the Haitian children born to illegitimate Haitian parents were illegals.

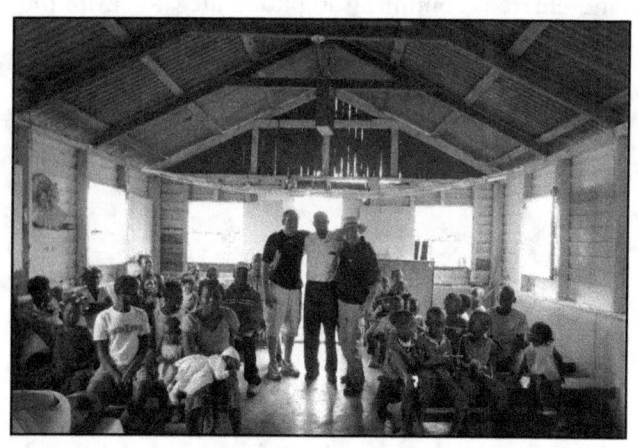

Dr. Stephen Simonetti and I in 2012

CHAPTER 17

Mission Trip to Haiti and Dominican Republic, March 2012

I am the founder and president of Mission Life International. I was joined by a team of twenty-two chiropractors who arrived in Haiti to serve chiropractic in March 2012. They served in a land where there are thousands of orphans roaming the streets. The roads in Haiti are paved with garbage and thousands of homeless people.

The chiropractors served in Haiti for four days, and then we traveled to Dominican Republic. On March 28, 2012, we were joined by fifty-one more chiropractors and students as they arrived in the jungles and remote villages of Dominican Republic. The mission chiropractors brought the healing power of chiropractic to hundreds upon hundreds of Haitians in the cities of Ouanaminthe and Cape Haiti. The blessed hands continued with thousands of adjustments in multiple Dominican Republic cities, villages, and hilltop towns. Continuing to respond to critical needs in Haiti, each chiropractor brought two suitcases filled with toothpastes, toothbrushes, soaps, shampoos, pencils, and small notebooks for the children. More than seven thousand pounds of items that we take for granted in the United States were distributed to children in lands where these goods were so desperately needed.

I was (and still am) the World Chiropractic Alliance NGO representative to the United Nations, which enabled me to attract a lot of people to my mission trips. This was my twentieth chiropractic mission trip to Haiti since the devastating January 2010 earthquake. I continue to focus attention on Haiti and inspire action that is making a meaningful difference in the lives of the Haitian people. We are making slow but steady progress in the most impoverished nation in the western hemisphere.

One of the chiropractors on this mission trip, Dr. Steve Simonetti, reported of his time in Haiti,

> The trip started on Saturday evening. We began with a team of twenty-two chiropractors. Dr. Morgan rented a bus and hired a driver. We then made the four-hour journey from the Santiago, DR, airport to Ouanaminthe, Haiti. One of Dr. Morgan's practice members, Boss Massel, joined us on the trip. He is a famous actor in Haiti and is personal friends with the President of Haiti.

Alex Thoni runs the orphanage founded by Dr. Morgan, and he met us at the border. During our trip, not only did I meet with the governor of the Ouanaminthe region, I also got to adjust him. Dr. Morgan recently moved the orphanage from Port au Prince to Ouanaminthe. The governor was very helpful and cannot wait to get adjusted again.

Humbly, each day after four o'clock, we would cross the border and stay in a small town in Dominican Republic called La Vejia, DaJabon. We stayed in family homes owned by relatives of some of my New York City chiropractic practice members. We had three chiropractic missionaries in each house. I paid for Dominican moms to go to the supermarket, and every morning and evening we would eat together in the town hall for breakfast and dinner. We usually had forty to fifty people at each meal.

In this town, the horses were not tied down, two hundred cows passed by every hour, and herds of sheep passed every two hours. We adjusted everyone in town as well as all the people they brought from other towns.

Every night my good friends Steve Simonetti, past president of the Congress of Chiropractic State Associations, and Gary Deutchman, founder of the Scoliosis Care Foundation, would teach the Thompson technique, scoliosis early detection, and other basic chiropractic adjusting techniques.

Each morning we would drive the bus into Haiti and adjust all the orphans throughout the city. We visited five different orphanages and adjusted about two thousand people per day at three different churches. Boss Massel then left to Port au Prince to meet with the President of Haiti. We were making every effort to get the government of Haiti to assist us in the opening of the first Christian chiropractic school. We already had the land, we just needed the finances.

We also helped our friends in La Vejia, Dominican Republic through our project called "Friends of La Vejia." There were many Haitian immigrants in this small Dominican-Haitian border village, where native locals had opened their homes and their hearts. If the Haitian children did not learn how to speak Spanish by their sixth birthday, they would be denied an education and forced to live on the street to fend for themselves. La Vejia needed a daycare center that would also provide Spanish language instructions.

The community, knowing that we had been blessed with healing hands, sensed that we had also been blessed with healing hearts and asked for our help. A young chiropractic student named Boo Burnier had raised one thousand five hundred dollars for the mission and chose to use these funds to get this project off the ground. Boo Burnier is the son of the world-renowned chiropractor Arno Burnier, DC.

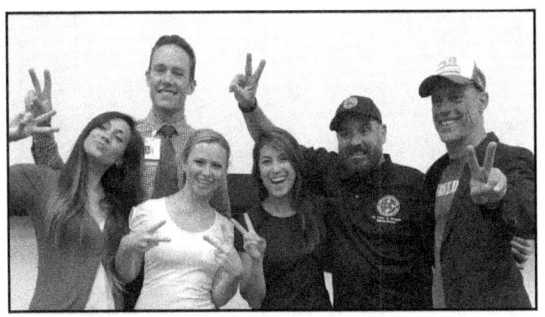

On this day we recruited 75 new members to the International Chiropractic Association.

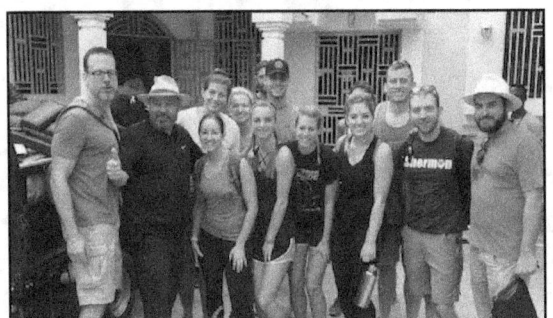

Joe McAulliffe, DC and Carlos Casinova, DC were the two doctors that helped all these chiropractic students during this mission trip.

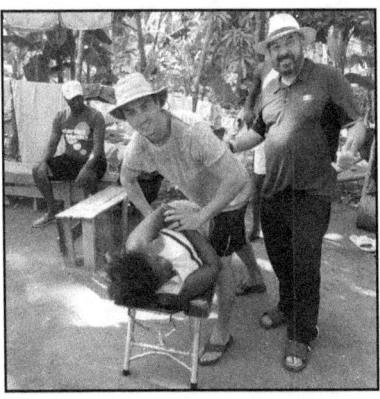

Daniel Fallu, DC adjusting in the village of Malfeti, Haiti.

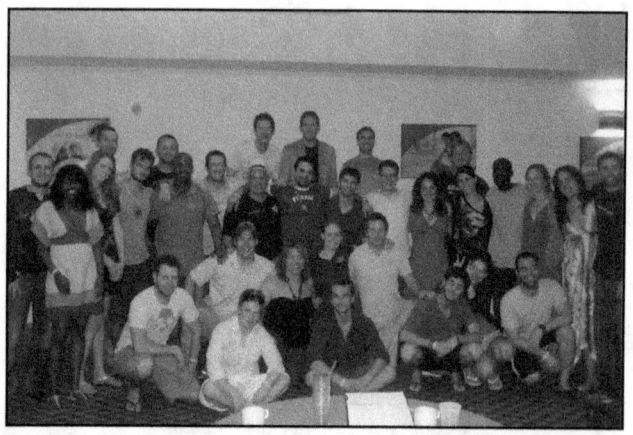
Our Missionary team in Puerto Plata, Dominican Republic in 2011.

CHAPTER 18

Mission Trip to Dominican Republic, October 2012

In October 2012 we had fifty-five chiropractic missionaries staying at a four-star all-inclusive hotel for four nights and five days. The hotel was on a gorgeous white sand beach with huge mountains behind it. Every night we shared in chiropractic philosophy and taught and reviewed chiropractic technique. We arose each morning at seven, ate breakfast, and were out the door serving by seven thirty.

We rented two buses and three SUVs to reach our twenty destinations. Our large chiropractic mission team was divided into smaller teams. Each team went to a school in the morning and a church in the afternoon. We ate together each night, sharing the miracles we witnessed during the day.

The previous July we had fifty chiropractic missionaries, and in January we had forty-five chiropractors serving chiropractic in schools, churches, nursing homes, police stations, and community centers. In the weeks before we arrived, we hired a group of dedicated Dominican chiropractic advocates to tell people the chiropractic story. We were on TV and radio days before we arrived. I told the chiropractic story to fifty pastors and priests throughout the North Coast of Dominican Republic. When we arrived at the churches, thousands of people were lined up waiting to be adjusted. At the schools, we taught Straighten Up America, and we checked approximately 250 children.

Each team saw about five hundred people a day—a total of five thousand people a day—for four days. (In Haiti, we usually have a small team of ten chiropractors, and they usually see over three thousand people a day.) We not only checked and adjusted the people, we told the chiropractic story to groups of fifty at a time. This was some awesome and fun work, and we were giving for the sake of giving, giving out of our own abundance. We were using the blessing that God bestowed upon us: our healing hands. It is the law of give and receive.

On this mission trip we had forty-eight chiropractic team members plus many Dominican chiropractic advocates. We were divided into ten chiropractic teams, and we spread the word of chiropractic throughout the North Coast of Dominican Republic. We focused on the correction and detection of vertebral subluxations. We also taught Straighten Up America at the forty schools we visited. We adjusted thousands of children on this magnificent chiropractic occasion.

We sent several chiropractic teams to Santiago on multiple occasions. I arrived a number of days early and had a chance to work in all three of our chiropractic offices. When I arrived in Santiago, I was told that we had an interview set up the coming Tuesday at a baseball stadium. Tuesday morning I decided to hike, eat, and meditate at Camp David. Innate merged with Universal very easily at this is location. It was a beautiful hotel and restaurant on the top of a huge mountain that overlooked the city of Santiago.

Innate told me to be extra early on this special day. The stadium was only a few minutes from our Las Collinas office and fifteen minutes from our three-bedroom apartment and chiropractic office. My meeting with Alexandra was scheduled for three fifteen, and we were to leave at that time from our office for the interview at the stadium. I wanted to be an hour early so we could tour around the stadium while we were waiting.

I arrived in the Santiago home office at two thirty, and Alexandra was already there. She told me that she had to go home and change her clothes and that she would be back in thirty minutes. At three o'clock, lightning started and went on for fifteen minutes. It was the closest that I had ever been to lightning. I said to myself that this was a message from God that we were going to be the chiropractors for Dominican Republic baseball team.

It started pouring, and Alexandra arrived back at the office at three thirty. We immediately jumped into my huge 4-wheel drive jeep. We drove down the road, and the streets were all flooded. Cars were drowning. The traffic was incredible. Every street was blocked off. I could not even move for a while. It was now 4:20; so much for my message from God. Luckily, I had rented this awesome vehicle. I started driving on the sidewalks. I was driving through the floods and passing the drowned cars.

We arrived at the stadium at exactly four thirty. We went into the reception room, sat down, and at that moment, the president of the Las Aguilas baseball team arrived. So much for Dominican time. He apparently uses US time. I told our baseball friend the chiropractic story in Spanish. He let me finish and then said in perfect English, "Why aren't you explaining this to me in English?" and then started laughing.

He asked me to take a picture of him with Alexandra. He gave me his camera, put his arm around her, and told her how good-looking she was. After the photography and flirting session was over, he said that he knew all about chiropractic and that he knew several US players who utilize chiropractic. "I am extremely interested," he said. "I need to bring this to my board and to the medical director of the team. We will have a phone conference with the medical director."

I spoke about one of the chiropractors who worked with us in Peru. Nick Necak, DC, was the chiropractor for the Peruvian Olympic team and had experience working with the Colombian Olympic team. Needless to say, God indeed had a very important message for me. "Be early, and tell the chiropractic story."

Thank you, Universal Intelligence, for all your blessings.

Record Holders Republic
Registry of Official World Records

A Governing Body for World Record Holders & Record Breakers

| Home | News | Search | Record Holders | Speed Darts | RHR TV | Certificates | Submit a Record | Contact us |

Peter Morgan

<< Back

Chiropractic (Chiromission)

Records

Record for **Peter Morgan** are displayed below:

Record Name	Record Description
Chiropractic Adjustments	Chiropractic Adjustments: 8 Days: 75,145. Peter Morgan, DC (Team Leader). In January 2013 Peter H. Morgan, DC armed with 38 chiropractors, 48 chiropractic assistants (students) and 22 volunteers, 75,145 patients (ages 2 months to 102 years) were cared for over a eight day period throughout the Dominican Republic and Haiti.
Chiropractic Care	Chiropractic Care: Most Patients: 2 Days: 21,545. Fran Capo. On April 4th and 5th, 2008, RockMetv host, Fran Capo and cameraman, Jeff Cobelli, volunteered to document the humanitarian world record efforts of Chromission.org in the Dominican Republic. Armed with a group of 28 chiropractors, 31 chiropractic assistants and 5 volunteers, which included the host and cameraman, 21,545 patients (ages 6 months to 98 years old) were cared for over a two-day period throughout the Dominican Republic and Haiti. Chiromission, which was founded by JC Doornick, Todd Herold and Peter Morgan, broke into teams and went into orphanages, jails, churches, schools and village streets to volunteer their services.
Chiropractic Mission Team	Chiropractic Mission Team: 108 members. Peter Morgan, DC (Team Leader). In January 2013 38 chiropractors, 48 chiropractic assistants (students) and 22 volunteers. A team of 108 cared for over 75,000 people throughout the Dominican Republic and Haiti.
Chiropractic Mission Trips	Chiropractic Mission Trips: 80. In August 2013 Peter H. Morgan, DC, lead his 80th international chiropractic mission.

RHR PRESIDENTS LISTED ON RECORD HOLDERS SECTION

General Info & Updates | Links | Trophies | Advisory panel | BOAR | About RHR | Designed and developed by Unicorn Designers

CHAPTER 19

World Record Mission Trip to Haiti, January 2013

Three years after the devastating earthquake that destroyed the capital city of Port au Prince, Haiti, we went on a mission trip with a chiropractic team of sixty-eight, comprising twenty chiropractors, thirty chiropractic students, and eighteen volunteers. Our volunteers were spouses with children and Christian missionaries. We stayed at the United Nations military base in Ouanaminthe, Haiti and were going to serve in hospitals, community centers, and factories.

We left for Puerto Plata to meet the other fifty chiropractors and students that were joining our chiropractic missionary team. Our team of sixty-eight in Haiti grew to a team of 108 in Dominican Republic. That night, a Wednesday, we had our first philosophy meeting with instrumental and motivational speakers

Bradley Rauch, Ron Sinagra, and me. The following morning our team of 108 were divided into twenty different teams and placed on four buses. Each team had a translator from the local English school, and we had a team coordinator at each site.

On Thursday and Friday mornings we adjusted in schools. Every school had between four hundred and a thousand students, teachers, and bus drivers. We averaged seven hundred adjustments at each school. In total, we checked and adjusted approximately fourteen thousand children on Thursday and the same number on Friday.

At the school I was serving, I asked the principal if we could adjust the parents when they came to pick up the students. He replied that normally we could, but that day they had a large conference with a hundred teachers attending. My next question was, "Can I give a chiropractic talk during the teachers' conference?" After a few phone calls, the answer was a resounding *yes*. I delegated this task to an outstanding chiropractic student named Sebastian Colon. After his presentation, we booked twenty-five schools for our next mission trip. In another school, one of our chiropractors taught Straighten Up America to over five hundred students, teachers, administrators, and parents.

In the late afternoons, we adjusted at churches and community centers. We indeed brought chiropractic to the masses. We met with the senator of the Puerto Plata region and the mayor of Sosua. Mission Life

International is our registered chiropractic non-profit organization in the United States and in Haiti. On that trip I signed the papers for our new Dominican Republic non-profit humanitarian organization, so now we have non-profit status in three countries. We are indeed international.

On this mission, we set our third world record for the number of patients adjusted. Our fourth world record is for the size of our chiropractic mission team. Over a period of eight days, our team of thirty-eight chiropractors, with the assistance of forty-eight chiropractic students, and twenty-two volunteers adjusted 75,145 people aged from two months to 102 years.

One of those people whom we adjusted on this trip was a blind man who can now see. Dr. Ron Sinagra performed a simple act of compassion, a chiropractic adjustment, on a totally blind person, and the man's life was changed forever. After his adjustment, the man's eyes became watery and he began to see shadows. The chiropractic students and the other people who were waiting to get adjusted witnessed this event.

During the Haitian part of our trip, we stayed in local people's homes. During the Dominican Republic part of our trip, we stayed at a five-star hotel with over 1,500 employees. They have their own heliport, a harbor filled with yachts, and the biggest waterfront casino on the island. While we were there we arranged for every employee to get checked and adjusted on our next trip. It was amazing that just a few miles away from this incredible beachfront resort lay a land of immense poverty.

To help with the language barrier, the mission chiropractors had help from twenty translators, who delivered the chiropractic story to educate the people as they waited. Chiromissions was able to share in this joy as the fruits of our labor began to show. We have been tremendously blessed by God to be born in the United States, and our greatest blessing of all is our gift of the healing hands. What our chiropractic missionaries received from the experience in Ouanaminthe was beyond words. The missionaries related, "We went to Haiti with one purpose: to give ourselves. We will never forget this!"

Back in Dominican Republic, the twenty teams were stationed all over the country. Many of the chiropractors were on their first mission trip, but they all prepared for an incredibly powerful week of love and service giving God's greatest gift to man. Chiropractic was shared with many people who may not have otherwise ever had the opportunity to experience a chiropractic adjustment.

Teams were located in mountain villages, city ghettos, orphanages, nursing homes, prisons, baseball fields, and villages on the tops of mountains. Most teams adjusted as many as a thousand people a day. The average team adjusted six hundred people a day. Almost every team adjusted every student in each local school.

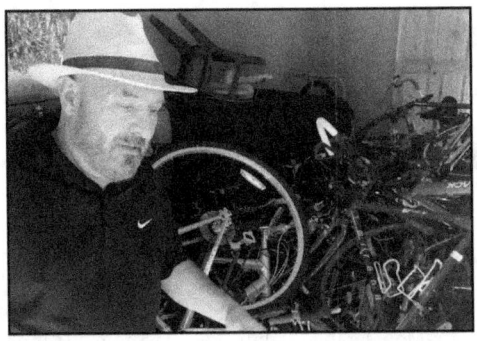

Chris Perrone, DC and the Mahopac Rotary club donated and shipped 75 bicycles to Ouanaminthe, Haiti.

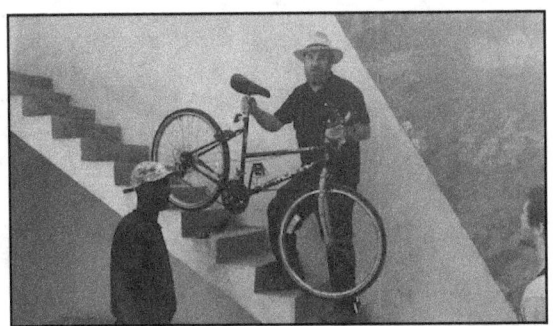

The bicycles arrived!

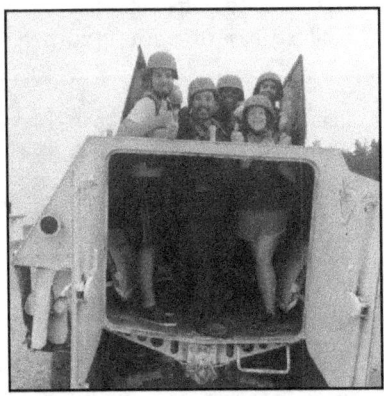

We stayed at the United Nations military base in Fort Liberty, Haiti for 25 different mission trips. The soldiers took us in their vehicles including some tank rides.

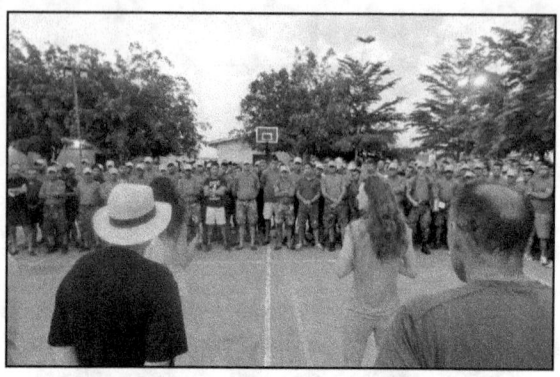

Dr. Montseratte Vilahur Gies, Dr. Simonetti and I teaching straighten up to 600 United Nations Military 2013 Ft. Liberte, Haiti

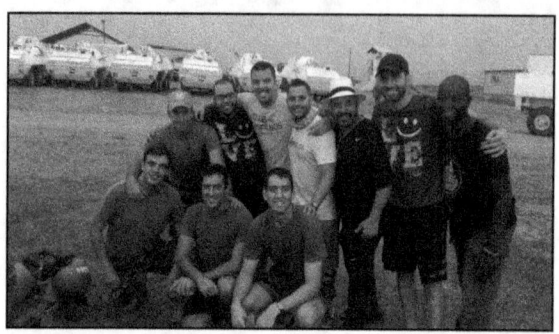

One of our teams at the UN Military base in Ft. Liberte, Haiti. 2017. We had 25 different teams stay at the Military base from 2013 to 2017.

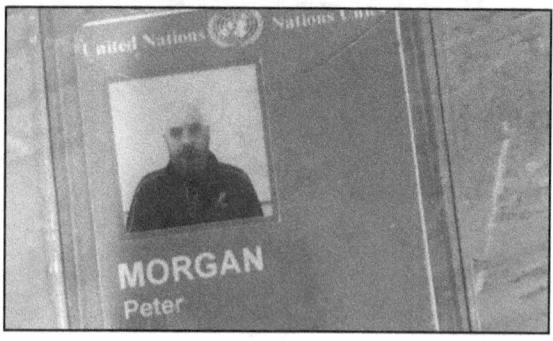

I have been the WCA Chiropractic Representative to the United Nations Department of Public information from 2010 to present (June 2020)

CHAPTER 20

The United Nations Military Base, Haiti, April 2013

Mission Life International runs an orphanage in Ouanaminthe, Haiti, that is 100 percent supported by chiropractors and their families and friends. The orphanage houses fifty children as well as support staff and provides schooling for fifty more children from the area. The school is across the street on a piece of property donated to the foundation. It is a covered outdoor structure with benches, desks, and black boards.

In April 2013 a group of us visited the United Nations military base, located approximately fifteen minutes from the orphanage. At that time there were 560 troops in the barracks, with trucks and a lot of rifles. The base was operated and manned by troops from Uruguay and Peru.

As the United Nations NGO/DPI chiropractic representative, I felt it would be good to meet with the commander of the base and inform him of our chiropractic mission work in Haiti. We were greeted by Col. Raul Passarino, who had received chiropractic care from one of only three chiropractors in Uruguay. Fortunately, we had brought our Astralite portable chiropractic adjusting tables.

We set up our tables and adjusted the commander and the captain of the base. The power of the adjustments superseded any conversation we had previously had. We then agreed to adjust all of the troops on our next mission trip a couple months later. The commander then made us an incredible offer: the United Nations military base would provide room and board for all of our chiropractic missionaries for a nominal fee. The base had air-conditioned barracks with bunk beds, television sets, tennis and basketball courts, a handball court, fully equipped air-conditioned weight lifting rooms, and an outdoor bar with a dance floor and pizza ovens. It was an oasis in the middle of a poverty-stricken desert.

Over the next four years we brought more than a thousand chiropractors on twenty-five mission trips at this base. Every nine months all military troops at the base would ship out and new soldiers would move in. Over those four years we met and adjusted five commanders, five colonels, five majors, many captains, and about 2,500 United Nations military personnel. Our missionaries also competed with the UN military in basketball, tennis, volleyball, soccer, and running. We never lost a basketball game, but we never won a soccer game, either.

All of the military bases in Haiti closed down in May 2017, and all United Nations personnel pulled out of Haiti in June of that year. As they left, the base was kind enough to donate thirty bunk beds for our children at the orphanage.

I wrote the following letter to Col. Raul Passarino, Urubatt 2 Commander.

Dear Col. Passarino,

It was a pleasure meeting you three weeks ago. Thank you so much for your hospitality. I am writing to confirm our arrival to your Urubatt UN base with our team of chiropractors on Sunday, June 23, 2013 at four o'clock. We will be in Haiti from Sunday through Tuesday, leaving on Wednesday for Dominican Republic. Our team currently consists of forty-eight people. I anticipate a team of approximately fifty-five. When we spoke I thought our team would be approximately twenty-five. Can you accommodate a larger team at your base? I could divide our team and put thirty at our orphanage and twenty-five at the Urubatt UN base. Let me know what you think. Again, thank you for your hospitality.

Peter H. Morgan, DC;
President, Mission Life International

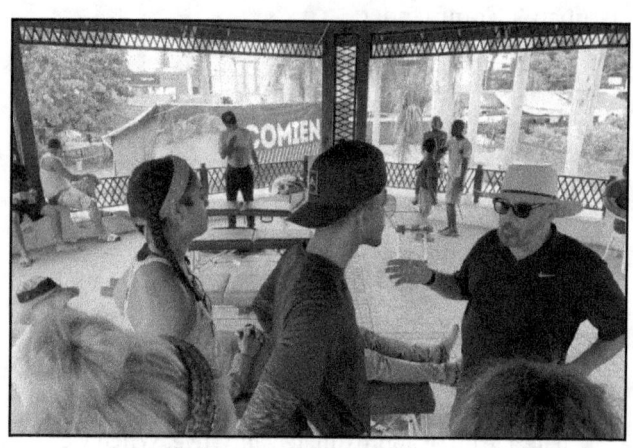

Dajabon, Dominican Republic 2019

CHAPTER 21

Mission Trip to Haiti, March 2018

In March 2018 we still had children who were orphaned or abandoned after the earthquake. They were the most awesome kids one could ever imagine. There were eight or nine kids that were now fifteen and sixteen years old. We had taken them in eight years before, when they were just seven or eight years old. They now help on every mission trip.

Junior drives one of our two three-wheeled vehicles. Raymonson also drives and speaks English. Edmonson has multiple talents and is our best soccer player. He scored three goals during our last game. Samuel is our DJ for our parties, and Liebenson plays multiple musical instruments: harmonica, flute, trumpet, clarinet, and saxophone. All the kids can sing and dance wonderfully.

They all live in our Mission Life Home, where they are integrated into a loving family environment. They are nurtured and supported in a Haitian family home. Strong bonds have developed within our Mission Life family, and even after the children are grown and leave Mission Life, these family relationships will endure.

The children have had the benefit of growing up in a stable, loving family environment that includes the necessities of life, such as clothing, meals, chiropractic healthcare, and a high-quality education. Our children will remain in the Mission Life Home until they are prepared to create lives for themselves as independent adults. Our home is a role model for the community in terms of quality caregiving, education, and chiropractic healthcare, and aims to be fully integrated into the larger community, not isolated from it.

We are currently constructing buildings for more children, housing for our missionaries, and an outdoor restaurant so that all our children have jobs. We also are working on creating jobs for our twenty translators.

In October 2017 I bought a used school bus and took it to the New Beginnings chiropractic seminar, where I am a frequent speaker. The attendees of the seminar filled our bus with contributions. Dr. Chris Perone and the rotary club donated seventy-five new and almost new adult bicycles for our "Love Cycles for Haiti" program. We received over three thousand pairs of new and almost-new shoes for our "Love Shoes for Haiti" program. My favorite program is our "Love Notes for Haiti" music program; we have nine guitars, three cellos, three violins, three flutes, two trumpets, two ukuleles, a saxophone, a clarinet, and a harmonica.

A few years ago I was watching the television

program *60 Minutes* one Sunday. The reporter was interviewing a musician who was running an orphanage in Paraguay. Astonishingly, this music teacher would go out to garbage dumps with many children and collect materials to make a variety of musical instruments. This music instructor then taught all the children how to play the instruments, and the children became phenomenal musicians. Incredibly, the children came to New York to play with a symphony orchestra at Carnegie Hall. They raised several million dollars for the construction of a new school.

I can't make musical instruments out of garbage, nor am I a music teacher, but I can create, so I developed the "Love Notes for Haiti" program. People donate all sorts of musical instruments, which I deliver to Haiti. I subsequently hire music teachers. Our children are awesome singers, incredible dancers, and now they play musical instruments. These young artists perform in the shows that we deliver on the last day of each mission trip. I surprisingly have even become a choreographer, and we have six performances a year.

Our family approach in the Mission Life Home is based on four principles: every child requires a family; children grow up most naturally with brothers and sisters; every child grows up in their own house within a supportive home environment; every child is provided a strong, vitalistic education taught by chiropractors.

We enable children to live according to their own culture and religion and to be active members of the community. We help them to recognize and express their individual abilities, interests, and talents. We ensure that children receive the education and skills training they need to be successful and contributing members of society. We share in community life and respond to the social development needs of society's most vulnerable children and young people. We establish facilities and programs that aim to strengthen families and prevent the abandonment of children. We join hands with community members to provide education and chiropractic health care, and teach vitalistic principles.

We offer children a place to call home and space to heal. By keeping brothers and sisters together with a full time professional foster parent in an individual home, we rebuild a loving family life. Mission Life homes are a positive environment designed to help children reach their full potential, but the real strength of the home lies in the collective power of foster parents, staff, and the surrounding community to help children find new hope and trust.

With a stable home, caring siblings, and a loving foster parent, the children can have happy childhoods and grow into caring, responsible, self-supporting adults. It is our determination that 100 percent of all donations shall go into construction and related costs of building and supporting the orphanage. Volunteer labor often has been offered and shall be utilized to the fullest extent possible. We welcome contributions from all sources, large or small. We consider all donations as sacred money of which we are but steward.

In 2020, Mission Life International is one of the few remaining aid agencies providing lifesaving sanitation, hygiene, and vitalistic education for thousands of Haitians. Mission Life International has educated thousands of people on good health and disease-prevention practices such as effective hand washing and hygienic food preparation. We are currently finishing the construction of a free chiropractic health center and birthing center on our campus. Our mission trips have brought more than two thousand chiropractors to Haiti since the 2010 earthquake.

I have led and successfully completed almost one hundred mission trips. I have taught thousands of chiropractic students and doctors of chiropractic about life. Our teams adjusted and helped millions of people. We have supporting more than four hundred youth and families in their efforts to generate income. We have built latrines, showers, and safe water points. We have educated more than 100,000 people on how to prevent cholera and other diseases, and we continue to do these things.

What I am most proud of is the fact that from 2010 to 2012 Mission Life International reunited more than one thousand children with their biological families. From 2012 to 2020 we have provided a family to orphaned children. We have sheltered, clothed, fed, and educated twenty-nine wonderful children. This could not be possible without the love and extremely hard work of Alex Thoni. Thank you, Alex.

Hola de Santo Domingo Dominican Republic.

Yo soy muy divertida y contenta. Todo esta bien.

APPENDIX

Mission Statements

MISSION STATEMENT OF ADVANCING CHIROPRACTIC

To unite chiropractors desiring to protect and support the rights of all doctors of chiropractic to provide vertebral subluxation correction and of all people who choose to receive such care.

To advance and promote vertebral subluxation-centered chiropractic to all people, including the public, the media, legislators, and those directly or indirectly associated with the chiropractic profession.

To support evidence-based practice guidelines which protect the right of patients to receive chiropractic care for the analysis and correction of vertebral subluxations.

MISSION STATEMENT OF THE COUNCIL ON CHIROPRACTIC PRACTICE

In July 1995, the Council on Chiropractic Practice was established with the mission of "developing evidence-based guidelines, conducting research and performing other functions that will enhance the practice of chiropractic for the benefit of the consumer."

MISSION STATEMENT OF THE NEW YORK CHIROPRACTIC COUNCIL

The New York Chiropractic Council's mission is to direct people to the realization that healing comes from within; and that ultimately the promotion of health and wellness is superior to the treatment of disease.

MISSION STATEMENT OF DR. D.D. PALMER

DD Palmer created the art, philosophy, and science of chiropractic. Palmer's mission was chiropractic.

I believe, in fact know, that the universe consists of Intelligence and Matter. This intelligence is known to the Christian world as God. As a spiritual intelligence it finds expression through the animal and vegetable creation, man being the highest manifestation. I believe that this Intelligence is segmented into as many parts as there are individual expressions of life; that spirit, whether considered as a whole or individually, is advancing upward and onward toward perfection; that in all animated nature this Intelligence is expressed through the nervous system, which is the means of communication to and from individualized spirit; that the condition known as TONE is the tension and firmness, the renitency and elasticity of tissue in a state of health, normal existence; that the mental and physical condition known as disease is a disordered state because of an unusual amount of tension above or below that of tone; that normal and abnormal amounts of strain or laxity are due to the position of the osseous framework, the neuroskeleton, which not only serves as a protector to the nervous system, but, also, as a regulator of tension; that Universal Intelligence, the Spirit as a whole or in its segmented parts, is eternal in its existence; that physiological disintegration and somatic death are changes of the material only; that the present and future make-up of individualized spirits depend upon the cumulative mental function which, like all other functions, is modified by the structural condition of the impulsive, transmitting, nervous system; that criminality is but the result of abnormal nervous tension; that our individualized, segmented spiritual entities carry with them into the future spiritual state that which has been mentally accumulated during our physical existence; that spiritual existence, like the physical, is progressive; that a correct understanding of these principles and the practice of them constitute the religion of chiropractic; that the existence and personal identity of individualized intelligences continue after the change known as death; that life in this world and the next is continuous—one of eternal progression. . . .

Therefore, inasmuch as the light of life was revealed to me in order that I should enlighten the world, and as our physical health and the intellectual progress of the personified portion of the Universal Intelligence depend upon the proper alignment of the skeletal frame,

I feel it my right and bounden duty to replace any displaced portion thereof, so that our physical and spiritual faculties may be fully and normally expressed, thereby not only enhancing our present condition, but making ourselves the better prepared to enter the next stage of existence to which this earthly existence is but a preliminary, a preparatory step.

By correcting these displacements of osseous tissue, the tension frame of the nervous system, I claim that I am rendering obedience, adoration and honor to the All-Wise Spiritual Intelligence, as well as a service to the segmented, individual portions thereof—a duty I owe to both God and mankind.

—D.D. Palmer, *The Chiropractor*

About the Author

Dr. Peter H. Morgan is a traditional Chiropractor, who for the past 35 years has and continues to lead and teach chiropractors, students and the public about chiropractic. Dr. Morgan has a compelling vision to make a difference in this world. Dr. Morgan has been in private practice in NYC for over 35 years. His mission in life is to constantly help others innately create excellence in their health and life. Dr. Morgan teaches DD Palmer's vision to as many people as possible.

Dr. Morgan is the founder and president of Mission life International A-501(c) (3) Not-for-profit organization which provides free care to underprivileged children and people in third world countries. Mission Life International has served over 1,500,000 youngsters in this capacity. Mission Life International has built wells, installed water filtration systems and built desks and blackboards since the devastating earthquake in Haiti of 2010. Mission Life has completed much of the construction of a new non-profit chiropractic health center that will be opening soon. It will be the first chiropractic center in the country of Haiti. The outdoor restaurant is almost complete where we will employ our older children to work and learn business. We currently employ 20 people from Haiti who would not have a means to support themselves. Our education arm educated our 29 children at our Mission Life Orphanage and 49 children at a nearby school. MLI has completed much of the construction of the chiropractic health center. The outdoor restaurant is almost complete and will employ our children. We currently employ 20 people from Haiti who would not have a means to support themselves.

Dr. Morgan was one of the first chiropractors to open chiropractic offices in the Dominican Republic. Over the years Dr. Morgan opened 10 different non-profit offices in the Dominican Republic. He now plans to open the first chiropractic school in the Dominican Republic which will also be the first chiropractic school in the Caribbean. Plans are for 2021.

Dr. Morgan is the Founder and Executive Director of Mission Life International Family orphanage and Chiropractic Center Ouanaminthe, Haiti. During the period of January 2010 to January

2013 the MLI chiropractic orphanage placed over 1,000 Haitian children who became orphaned in the January 2010 earthquake with Haitian families who lost their own children. In June of 2012 we moved from Port Au Prince to Ouanaminthe, Haiti. We moved our children into better housing with a security guard and employed a nun to help provide structure in their daily routine and assist in their daily activities. Many of our older children are pursuing careers in trades and also helping our mission trips as translators. Mission Life International presently clothes, feeds and houses 29 children at the orphanage in Ouanaminthe, Haiti. Dr. Morgan takes hundreds of people each year to visit the orphanage. Mission Life International has constructed 4 buildings in Ouanaminthe, Haiti.

Dr. Morgan is founder and president of ChiroMissions with the purpose is to promote chiropractic and adjust all those who are subluxated throughout the world, especially in developing countries where resources are terribly limited. Dr. Morgan has led 99 chiropractic mission trips to developing nations and his next trip will be December 26, 2020-Jan. 3, 2021. On October 30, 2020 Life University (largest chiropractic school in the world) awarded Dr. Morgan as the 2020 Chiropractor of the Year.

Dr. Morgan believes no woman or baby should die during childbirth. Haiti has the highest maternal and infant mortality rate in the westernhemisphere. Nearly all maternal and infant deaths in Haiti are preventable with access to a skilled birth attendant. Dr. Morgan wants to make childbirth safer in Haiti. His mission is for all women of Haiti to have access to skilled prenatal, postnatal and delivery care while simultaneously receiving necessary complementary skilled chiropractic care. Dr. Morgan has created the vision for a birthing Center that will provide a safe place for Haitian women to receive compassionate and respectful care at the hands of skilled midwives and chiropractors. No woman will be turned away. We anticipate that every morning 50 women will start their day waiting to be seen by the midwives. When it's time to deliver their baby, women will now be able to do so with far greater safety in the sanctuary of the Mission Life International Birthing Center.

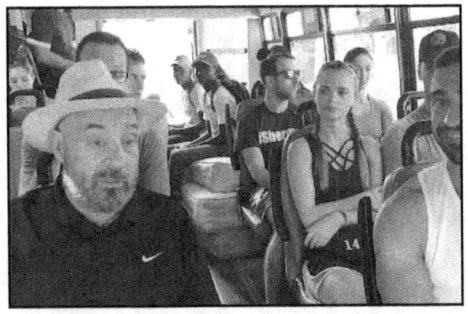

On this day Raymonson and Sedrack (boys I have known for ten years at the orphanage) became translators for our mission.

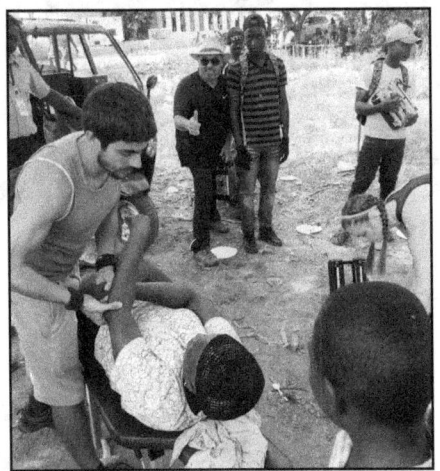

Leon Monzón, DC is one of the most extraordinary chiromissionaries I have ever met.

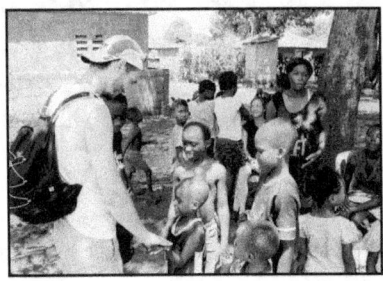

Time to take a break after adjusting hundreds of people.

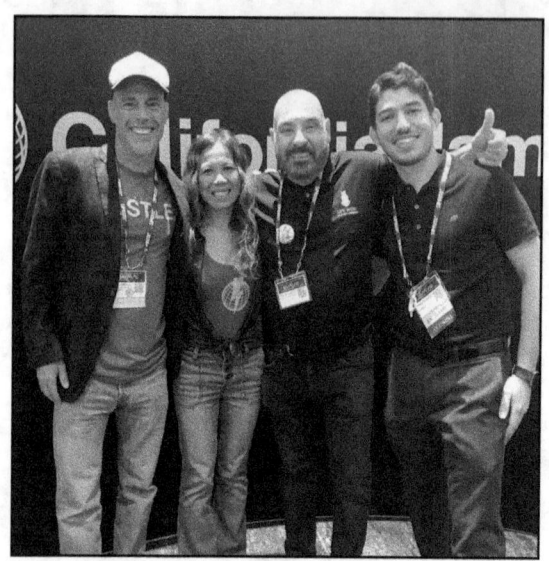

Loved my time at Cal Jam with Billy Demoss, DC.

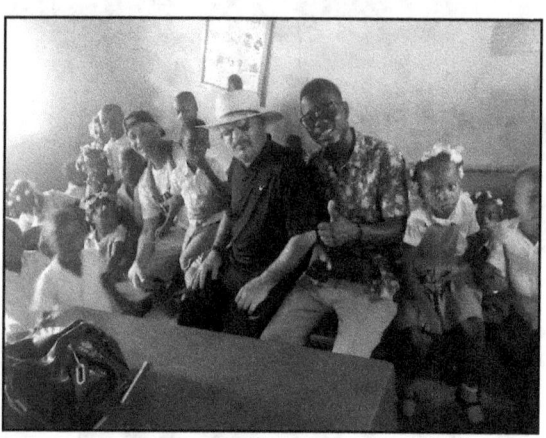

Henri, DJ Sammy and I having fun at a school. DJ Sammy, Henri Rosenblum, DC and I enjoying our visit to a school in Ouanaminthe, Haiti. Of course we checked all the kids.

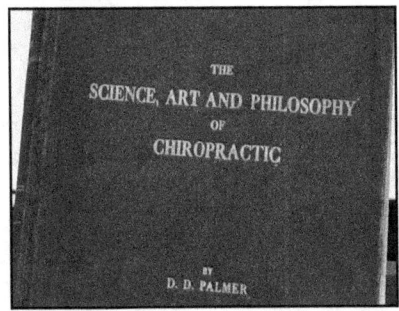

The first chiropractic book I bought that
I did not have to use for school.

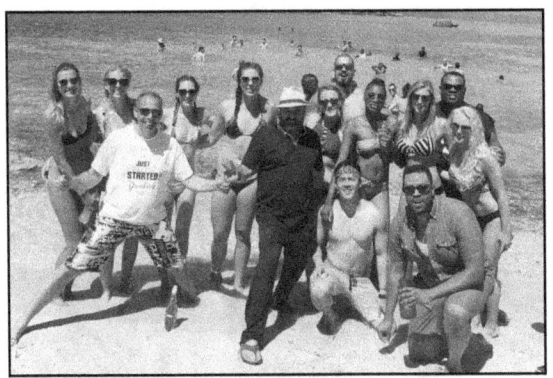

We had a team of 60 chiropractors on this
trip to the beach in Labadee, Haiti.

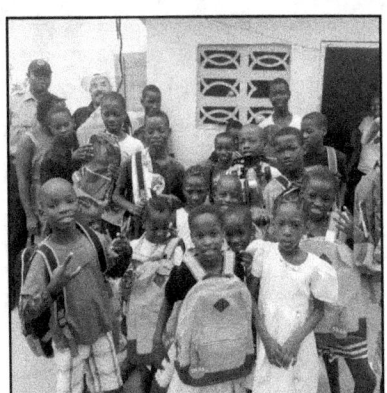

Backpack day at the Mission Life
International family orphanage.

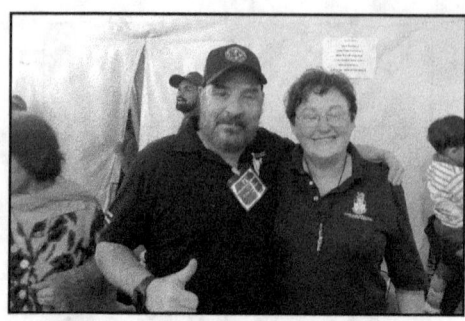

Mission trip to India with Lynn McAvenia, DC. Lynn told the chiropractic story to thousands of people each day.

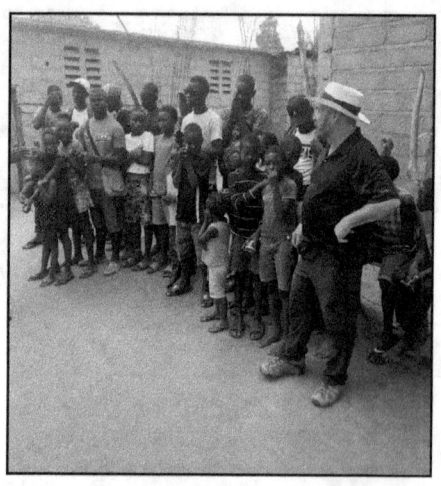

Our kids from the Mission Life orphanage went on a field day with me.

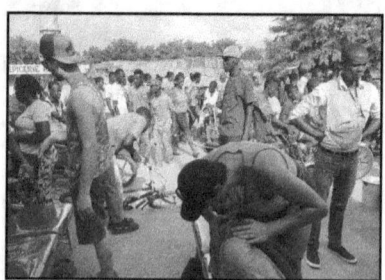

Outside the Codevi factory. 18,000 employees pass by this spot between 4 and 6 PM on working days.

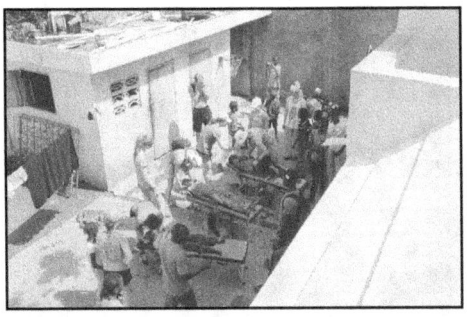

Our old orphanage in Ouanaminthe, Haiti. Our security guard Joseph now lives there.

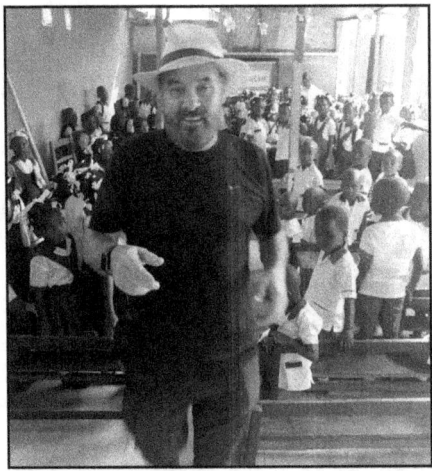

I love visiting our children's school.

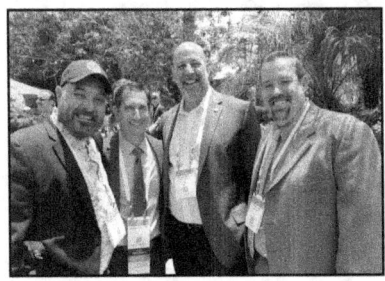

Brian Stenzler, DC President California Chiropractic Association; Ron Oberstein, DC President Life West Chiropractic College and Bharon Hoag, executive Director of One Chiropractic at the California Chiropractic Association Convention.

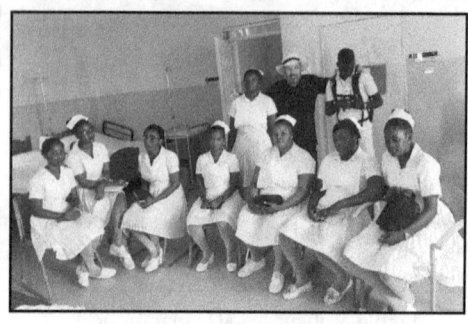

I adjusted all of these Nurses at Univers Hospital, Ouanaminthe, Haiti.

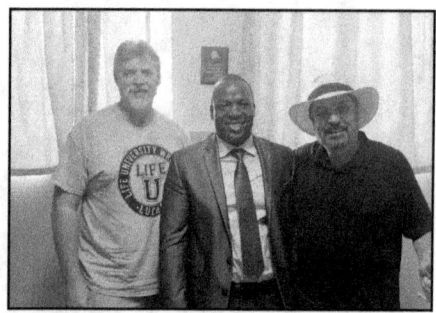

Robert Scott, DC President of Life University, Dr. Lesly Manigat Medical Director of Univers Hospital and I at Univers Hospital.

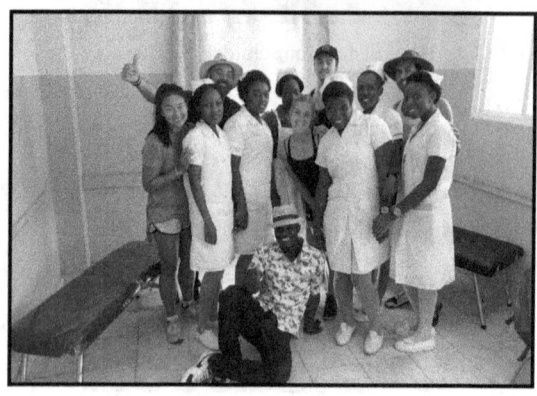

Clara White, DC Veronica Gobeil, DC Daniel Fallu, DC and Samuel Garcon adjusting the staff at Univers Hospital.

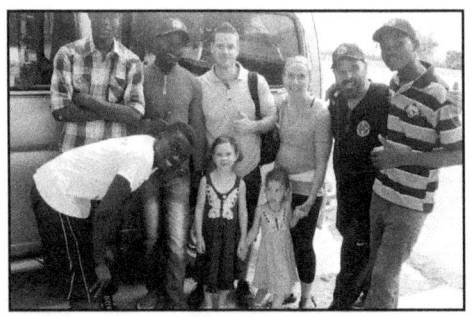

Dan Sullivan, DC with his family in Cap-Haitien, Haiti. 2015.
Mednightson, Sammy DJ and Sammy Garcon.
Amanda Sullivan was 22 weeks pregnant.

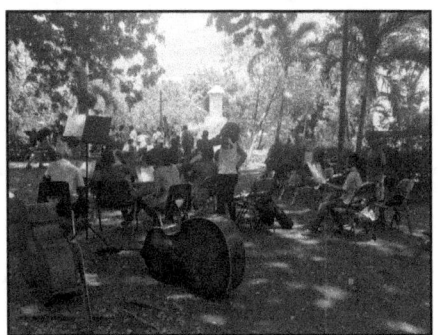

Our Love notes for Haiti program is taking off.

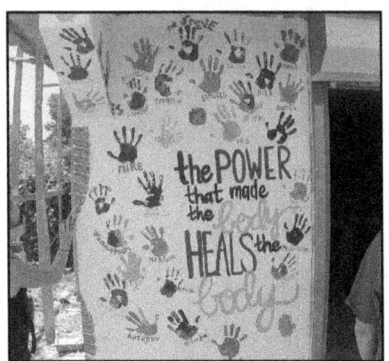

One of the walls of our Kitchen building in Ouanaminthe, Haiti.